© Nicole Goddard

About the Author

JASON MULGREW is a self-proclaimed "Internet Quasi-Celebrity" whose blog, Everything Is Wrong with Me: 30, Bipolar, and Hungry, has received more than 200 million hits since its inception. Originally from Philadelphia, he now lives in New York City, where he works for a white-shoe law firm that tolerates his blue-collar ways.

EVERYTHING
Is **Wrong**
with ME

EVERYTHING Is Wrong with ME

A Memoir of an American Childhood Gone, Well, Wrong

JASON MULGREW

HARPER ● PERENNIAL

NEW YORK ● LONDON ● TORONTO ● SYDNEY ● NEW DELHI ● AUCKLAND

HARPER ● PERENNIAL

The names and identifying characteristics of some of the individuals featured throughout this book have been changed to protect their privacy.

All photographs throughout are courtesy of the author unless otherwise stated.

EVERYTHING IS WRONG WITH ME. Copyright © 2010 by Jason Mulgrew. All rights reserved. Printed in the United States of America. No part of this book may be used or reproduced in any manner whatsoever without written permission except in the case of brief quotations embodied in critical articles and reviews. For information address HarperCollins Publishers, 10 East 53rd Street, New York, NY 10022.

HarperCollins books may be purchased for educational, business, or sales promotional use. For information please write: Special Markets Department, HarperCollins Publishers, 10 East 53rd Street, New York, NY 10022.

Designed by Mia Risberg

FIRST EDITION

Library of Congress Cataloging-in-Publication Data is available upon request.

ISBN 978-0-06-176665-7

10 11 12 13 14   OV/RRD   10 9 8 7 6 5 4 3 2 1

to my parents . . .
my god, i'm sorry

Acknowledgments

This book would not be possible without the help of several wonderful, talented, patient, and forgiving people (with special emphasis on those last two). Rakesh Satyal was given a series of run-on sentences and poop jokes and made it—dare I say—beautiful. Brian Saliba took a chance and (I hope) was rewarded. Likewise, Erin Malone and Joel Begleiter put their careers and quite possibly their lives on the line; I thank them for their loyalty, which I could not repay in a thousand lifetimes or two thousand beers (I am, however, contractually obligated to mention that they are the most attractive agents in the world).

My family was somewhat important in this process, providing me with ammunition—I mean, with research and background information—as well as pictures. Particular thanks go to John and Maureen Dawson. If it were not for their beach house, the cold of winter, and the good people who make Guinness, this project wouldn't have gotten past page three and I would likely be living out of my car right now.

Brendan Caffrey is a mad genius who has always made me look good, and Tina Concha and Danielle Del Vecchio literally helped me put this together. Thanks to many other friends who read and commented on various drafts, even if their comments were along the lines of "Are you serious with this? Like, this is what you want to hand in?"

Lastly, thanks and thanks galore to my mom Kathleen, dad Dennis, brother Dennis, and sister Megan. If you are reading this and are still speaking to me, we did good. If you are reading this, are still speaking to me, and are wearing really expensive jewelry and jetpacks, we did *real* good.

After creating a formula that combines the amount of alcohol involved, the number of years passed, the character/integrity of the protagonists, and my distaste for fact-checking, I have determined that the following is between 94 and 97 percent true. Thank you for your support.

Preface

Writing a book is a fantastical exercise in manic depression.

The highs, when they come, are magnificent. Throughout my life, I've rarely experienced such surges of adrenaline. I don't really play sports, mostly because they seem like a lot of work. I don't particularly care about my job, although it allows me to make lots of personal phone calls, because like many people my age I have forsaken inspiration for a steady paycheck. Nor do I do anything that I can be particularly proud of. Volunteering seems like a scam to me. (Work for free? Really?) I am not a member of any organizations, fraternities, or brotherhoods, because all the bonding creeps me out a little bit. And I have no children, or at least none that I care to acknowledge; I'm no Gregor Mendel, but when you mix Irish Catholic and Asian you're not supposed to get a child that looks like a Chinese Rudy Huxtable, so I'm not going to be the one to pay $450 a month.

Previously, my greatest accomplishment came when touring Europe as a college student several years ago. In one glorious stretch, I consumed so much alcohol, so many barbiturates, and so much *skinke** that my reckless behavior resulted in me peeing the bed in six European countries in a span of twenty-six days.** It was difficult, but I was determined. And I have a drinking problem, so that helped. And yes, I was single at the time (and as of this writing, still am).

Not to belittle my accomplishment, which was and will always be extraordinary, but the thrill I got from peeing in all those foreign countries does not compare to the rush of writing a book. I have learned that in the spectrum of adrenaline rushes, *creating* far surpasses *urinating*. There are moments in the writing process when all of your research, your outlines, and your preparation come together and you are just *doing* it. Your fingers work like pistons pummeling the keyboard and the words fly onto the page so quickly that it's hard to keep up. You zone out everything else and you just see it—the characters, alive; the setting, before your eyes; the story, just as you had experienced it; all the different words you can use for *poop,* preferential treatment given to the simple and effective *poo*—and it's magic. You'll even run out of beer but be so into the writing that you can't stop and won't stop to get another. So you'll scream at your roommate Brian to bring you one. When he doesn't, you'll realize it's because Brian moved out over two years ago and you no longer have a roommate. So maybe you don't need another beer. Slow down there, tiger.

---

* That's Danish for "ham." It will also be the name of my next pet.
** England, France, Spain, Italy, the Czech Republic, and Holland, if you're keeping score at home.

When you finally stop typing, you'll bolt up from your chair, your hands quivering, tears of joy streaming down your face, sporting a decent half erection because, really, it's a miracle you can even get a halfie going with your high blood pressure.* Then you'll read over what has just poured out of you and you'll say, "Yes, I have done it. I have fucking done it. I am a great writer. And I still need a beer." But because your roommate Brian is being a dick and still hasn't brought you one, you'll have to get it yourself. Or again, maybe it's because he moved out. A long, long time ago. Semantics. Probably should get some water instead.

These are the best times: You've written something that you're proud of and you can be happy, truly happy with yourself. The feeling is not unlike falling in love with someone new, but without all the nervousness and the sex. Actually, there may be sex involved for some writers, but there wasn't with me. Which sucked.

But sadly, these moments of intense joy are few and far between. They represent probably less than 1 percent of the book-writing experience, since it is hard to sustain such stretches of inspiration, especially when TNT is almost constantly running a *Law & Order* marathon. And when these fleeting instances of productivity escape, they are replaced by dark, dark times. Seconds of pleasure give way to hours of staring at a blinking cursor on the blank page, wondering where and how to begin. This is one of the most overwhelming and intimidating feelings a

---

* Really, sex for me nowadays is the rough equivalent of sticking a wet dishrag into a shotglass.

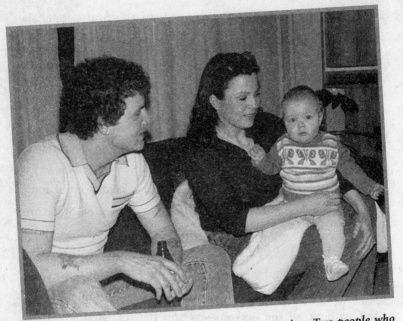

Three people who have very little concept of parenting. Two people who drank too much that night and later vomited because of it.

person can have, right up there with taking your driver's license test, or making a marriage proposal, or the first time you go to a gay club, or the first time you realize you like and possibly even *love* being at a gay club.

And when the moments of clarity are slow to come, self-doubt creeps in. The thoughts come at you in rapid succession: "What the hell am I doing? I'm not qualified to write a book! It took me a month and a half to find the *S* on the keyboard, so in most of my first draft I used *$* instead!" and "Why can't I figure this out? What the hell is wrong with me? How hard can it possibly be to throw my family under the bus so that I can buy a high-def TV and force them to cut off contact with me for the rest of my life?" and "Holy shit—I just realized that I haven't showered in four days! Something smells like hot-dog water and I think it's coming from my pants!" Sadness sinks you. Depression takes over. And the only thing you can do is get drunk, troll the Internet for sex, and hope it turns around.

I was warned that many first-time authors have difficulty with the enormity of the task of writing a book, so I tried to be prepared. I took a leave of absence from my full-time job to write this memoir, so I had plenty of time to record anecdotes from Little League, when I spent my time on the bench learning about sex from the older players (and no, not in that way).* I had months to write down the memories of those first few Christmas mornings when my dad would wince when I made a bigger deal about getting *Grease* on VHS than now owning "every single [expletive deleted] He-Man guy." Weeks and weeks to recollect the halcyon days when I was thin, mostly hairless, and handsome, those days that I miss so much when every Saturday night I look at myself in the shower and realize that yes, I, Jason Mulgrew, now a grown-ass man, look like a fucking bear when I'm naked.

No, the first task was to take stock of my life in the more immediate sense. Like a general in wartime, I looked at the situation, immersed myself in thought and cheap vodka, and came up with a battle plan. If I was going to write a good book, I needed to create the proper environment in which to write this book. Once I felt comfortable in the physical sense, the words would flow.

---

* Well, maybe a little.

I had to clean my room. My bedroom was where most of the writing would take place, and to be successful I needed to *feel* successful, to give the impression of success. I threw out all the empty beer cans and half-eaten mozzarella sticks that had accumulated on my desk over the past few months, as I needed a proper workspace. Then I turned my attention to the closet, which was a nest of such horror and depravity that I dare not speak of it in depth here, as I am just now getting over the night terrors it caused me (lesson: just because after you masturbate into an old pair of boxers you throw it into the depths of your closet, that doesn't mean that it magically disappears). Then I cried. Then I made the bed. Finally, I was done. And it only took two weeks.

Once my room was in tip-top shape, I turned my attention to the living room, which I decided needed a new furniture arrangement. I would say that this was an attempt to create an apartment more in line with feng shui, but I have no idea what feng shui is.* After several attempts, the discovery of two neatly rolled and nicely preserved joints, and four broken fingers, I settled on theater-type tiered sitting, with my loveseat in front of the larger couch in front of a few folding chairs. This process of trial and error took thirty-three days. Not a bad way to spend a month.

I felt like I was getting closer to the book. I would think about it a lot, often discussing it over drinks with friends or with strangers I met while vacationing in Mexico, Florida, Ha-

---

* Although I did once kiss a half-Filipina girl, so I'm pretty in tune with Asian culture. It was actually sort of a force-kiss, but, again, semantics.

waii, and Mexico again. I was so enamored with Mexico that during one of these trips I decided that as a side project to the memoir, I would write a history of the Oaxaca region. I figured that this side project, which would really be more of a fictional history due to my aversion to research, would help my ideas flow for this book. So I began preparations to begin work on this new

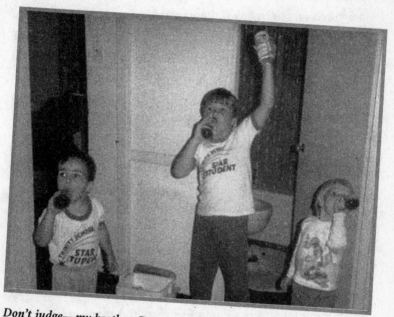

Don't judge—my brother, Dennis, and I were star students, so we could enjoy a cold one every once in a while. My cousin Lindsay, however . . . let's just say that she had her battles with the bottle.

endeavor, namely by writing a letter to my editor asking for an advance of at least $46,000 for "purposes of ensconnsing [*sic*] myself with the people, cultere [*sic*] and love of the people of

Mexico, and their cultere, [*sic*], and the love, and miscellaneius [*sic*] expenses related hitherto." But then I found another bottle of tequila under the floorboards of the little hut in which I was staying and, to be honest, I forget what happened over the next three or four days. I don't think I got around to that history, though, because I found the unsent letter to my editor when preparing my taxes the following year in the process of tracking down receipts to write off these trips as business-related.

Back in my apartment in New York City, the time for the book still had not yet come. Looking around the apartment, at my clean bedroom and my living room with the theater seating, I realized that my physical environs had been readied. And though I was very tan and healthy-looking in my complexion, I had been feeding on a steady diet of steak and expensive to semi-expensive alcohol since I had received my advance for this memoir. My body now softer than ever before, I followed the old axiom "Sound body, sound mind" and joined a gym. After all, now that I was writing full-time, free to make my own hours and no longer a nine-to-five slave to The Man, I figured I could spare an hour a day to get in shape. Exercising my body would help me exercise my mind, and when I accepted the Pulitzer Prize for this book in a few years, I'd thank my parents, my girlfriend Carmen Electra, and my trainer, Mercurio. Then Carmen and I would go have sex in the shower, and I would actually take off my shirt, no longer ashamed of my pudgy torso or growing quickly tired from both standing *and* thrusting at the same time. It would be wonderful.

But sadly, the gym did not last. I found the place to be too suffocating. Working out only made me tired and sweaty, and

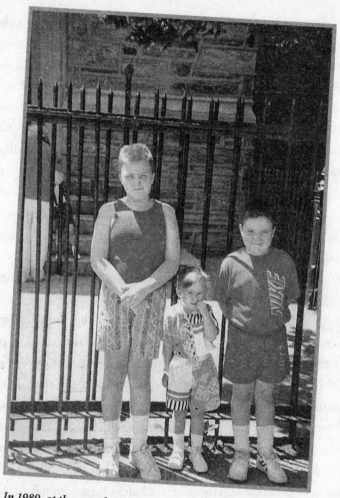

In 1989, at the age of ten, I went through a brief lesbian phase. Brief, but intense.

being around all those in-shape people hurt my self-esteem. And the last thing I needed when I was writing the story of my early life was low self-esteem (or rather, *lower* self-esteem). With nowhere else to turn, I looked outside myself for strength.

During this book-writing ordeal (really, there is no other word), I relied heavily on my friends. They helped me through my writer's block by taking me out, spending time with me, joining me for drinks, and allowing me to pay for all of it with my large and glorious book advance. I'd also pay for any people that came with my friends, especially if said people had nice boobies and/or daddy issues. This cost me thousands of dollars, but it was worth it. I felt good, happy. More important, I was on the way to changing literary history forever. Eventually.

Every week I'd get a call from my editor, who was always "just checking in." The calls followed a rote formula that went something like:

Editor: "Hey Jason. I'm just calling to check in. How's it going?"

Me: "Good, but I'm pretty tired. I was up until like five A.M. last night learning how to play the first Clapton solo from "Crossroads"—you know, the live version from *Wheels of Fire*. I think I have it down pretty good and am going to start on the second one, which is a little harder and longer than the first. Then this afternoon I went to brunch with Nicole, Annie, and Ben for like six hours, so after all the banana French toast and the vodka tonics, I'm pretty wiped out. But in two hours I'm going to pregame at Jeremy's place before we see Joseph Arthur tonight, so I'm thinking of taking a quick nap."

Editor: "Um, right. And how is the book coming?"

Jason: "Oh—that's coming along well. Really well, even. How's the book coming on your end?"

Editor: "Well, we're just sort of waiting for a manuscript from you and then we'll move from there. So . . ."

Jason: "Totally bro, I understand. I'll have something for you soon."

Editor: "Great. I'll give you a ring next week then."

Jason: "Perfect. Oh, one more thing—do you have a pot connection? I think my guy's in jail or dead or something because I can't get a hold of him."

Editor: [*silence*]

[This exchange more or less repeated itself every week for over three months. If I can give any advice to first-time writers, it's to be prepared to deal with your editors. They can be a major pain in the ass and occasionally entirely unreasonable.]

Eventually, I got up the gumption to ask my editor for those two little words that every writer adores: *ex-tension*. I had changed my environment, traveled, and (tried to) change myself physically, and through these trials it had become obvious that stress was the biggest obstacle for me. I figured that once the extension was granted, the stress would go away and the book would come easily. My editor sighed, then was silent for a few minutes, then sighed again, then said he'd think about it and get back to me in a few days. Content with myself and knowing that my request would be granted, I went to Cancun to get fucked up for a week.

When I came back four weeks later, I had several messages on my cell phone from both my editor and my agent. Since my editor sounded pretty upset about me "disappearing," as he called it, I decided instead to call back my agent, who sounded only slightly less upset than my editor did. Apparently, the publisher was pretty pissed off that I left the country and this was in bad faith and I was defaulting on my contract and yada

yada yada blah blah blah and my request for an extension was denied. The publisher came back with another two words that were much less pretty than the two I suggested: *law-suit.* So I decided to get writing.

What you hold in your hands right now is the result of sixteen days of blood, sweat, piss, more sweat, and tears. Sixteen days that were at once the best and worst of my life. Sixteen days that, most important, have passed.

This is my book. I hope you enjoy it, because I worked very hard on it. If not, well, that's fine, too. I mean, I wrote this thing in two weeks. Jerk.

EVERYTHING Is Wrong with ME

Chapter One

A Break,
a Beginning

It was the summer of 1973, a great time to be young, dumb, and in my father's case, full of Budweiser, Quaaludes, and reheated pizza. That lost generation—born too late to be hippies, too early to be disco freaks—strutted up and down the streets of my parents' South Philadelphia neighborhood, a grid of row-home-filled streets filled with working-class Irish Catholics and some Polish Catholics, bounded on the south by the Walt Whitman Bridge, the sports stadiums, and the Navy Yard; on the east by the mighty Delaware River; on the north by fancy Society Hill and, farther north, Center City; and on the west by the worst border of all: the Italian neighborhood that, thanks to *Rocky*, South Philly would become famous for in a few years. Sporting impeccable Afros and now-ridiculous but then-cool hairstyles—the men looking like Rod Stewart or Eric Clapton and the women like "Crazy on You"–era Ann or Nancy Wilson, but without all the trappings of fame and talent and good-looks—and in their hip clothes, members of that tween generation joined friends hanging out on the corner, drinking beers, and listening to Bad Company, Derek & the Dominoes, and Mott the Hoople. After getting done with work, there wasn't much to do aside from getting drunk and listening to music. Which was fine for just about everybody involved.

My dad, Dennis Mulgrew, had just graduated from St. John Neumann High School, on Twenty-sixth and Moore streets. He was tall and lean, slowly beginning to collect tattoos, and was without his trademark mustache that he would wear throughout my lifetime. He wasn't my dad at the time—he would be "blessed" with his firstborn six years later, one year after marrying my mom—but rather just some guy who liked to drink, chase women, listen to rock 'n' roll, work on cars, and look good. In short, your typical teenager, fresh out of high school, not quite ready to embark on adulthood, instead occupied with more pressing and immediate matters, all in some capacity relating to narcotics and/or pussy.

He had recently gotten a job on the waterfront in Philadelphia, where he and pretty much every guy he knew worked as a longshoreman,* but on the weekends during the summer my

---

* To this day, I'm not exactly sure what longshoremen do. I think it has something to do with taking cargo from ships that come into port on the Delaware River and putting half that cargo in warehouses and selling the other half to your friends on the cheap. Also, there is a lot of cursing, napping, drinking

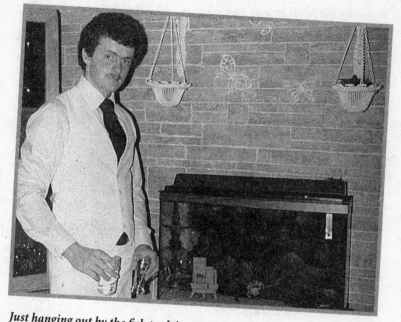

Just hanging out by the fish tank in a three-piece suit, jacket off, about to pour a can of beer into a little glass. You know, normal, everyday stuff.

dad would head "down the shore" to North Wildwood, a small island off the Jersey Shore, exit six on the Garden State Parkway, where his entire South Philadelphia neighborhood transplanted itself every year from Memorial Day to Labor Day.* There, in this quaint beach town filled both with large Victorians and kitschy and colorful motels, united by a miles-long boardwalk dotted with fudge and taffy shops, pizza parlors, and of course,

on the job, and complaining about your wife involved. I could be wrong, but I'm pretty sure that's the basic gist of it.

* Whether this is because North Wildwood had more bars per square mile than any other shore town in New Jersey is unknown, but presumed.

all the carnival games and rides, he shared a shore house with a dozen or so other guys from the neighborhood, guys with names like Franny, Billy, Frankie, and Mikey and nicknames like Shits, Tooth, Flip, and Porky. Neighborhood guys, solid guys, genuine guys; guys who had known each other since kindergarten, guys whose fathers had all grown up together, guys whose understanding of the world outside their neighborhood was limited to the names of things they were smoking (Acapulco Gold, black Afghani hash, Hawaiian indica, etc.).

On this Saturday afternoon in July of '73, my dad and his friends, being good blue-collar young men of Irish Catholic descent, were taking part in the preferred activity of their fathers and their father's fathers and their father's father's fathers before them: getting messed up and doing stupid shit. This could take various forms, such as:

- getting drunk and starting fights (usually with each other)
- getting high and stealing cars for joyrides
- taking some pills and breaking into friends' houses to steal household appliances and throw them in the ocean or bay
- something involving poop (human or animal)
- all of the above

Despite being a few months shy of his eighteenth birthday, my dad had made plans to spend that Saturday drinking with some friends from Third and Durfor, a corner hangout back in the city, at Moore's, a bar on the inlet that sat atop jagged rocks that jutted out into the Atlantic. But he was broke. The night before, he had loaned his buddy Charlie [pronounced *CHA-lee*] his last twenty dollars, which Charlie had promised to repay first thing Saturday [pronounced *SAH-ur-dee*] morning. But Charlie never showed up. So instead of going to Moore's, my father joined his friends in a much cheaper activity: jumping off the pier into the bay. That was the plan, at least. Never mind that they had been drinking (and probably doing other impairment-inducing things) since they had woken up. And never mind that the distance between the pier and the water below was not in-significant. And never mind that no one in their group had ever done this before. None of these facts was deemed a deterrent.

I'm not exactly sure about this, but I think that in the early '70s a man's manliness and testicular fortitude were symbolized by the pomposity of his hair. My dad was fortunate in this re-gard. The Mulgrew genes guaranteed that he and his four broth-ers sported the biggest and baddest white-boy Afros their side of Girard Avenue, huge auras of kinky hair that extended straight outward and upward, looking not like they had accidentally stuck their fingers in electric outlets and had been shocked, but rather like they *intentionally* stuck their fingers in sockets because they looked *that. fucking. good.* So when the group, now gathered on the dock, lingered there—looking over the water below them, tacitly waiting for someone to step forward and offer to make the first jump off the bulkhead into the green-blue deep below—his Afro firmly in place, possibly touching it up while Zeppelin's "Black Dog" blared on the radio, my dad happily volunteered.

Never much for oceanography (or really any *graphy*, except perhaps pornography), my dad didn't realize that as he was preparing to make his jump the waters of the bay were receding with the tide. He was aware of the existence of tides in general (probably), but at the moment he was more concerned with turning up the rock 'n' roll and "Boy, do Shelly's tits look great in that bikini" than the moon's gravitational effect on our oceans. Therefore, it probably didn't cross his mind, as he was taking off his shirt and pulling one last swill of beer, that the water below might not be very deep, possibly not deep enough to accommodate a diver, possibly not deep enough to accommodate a diver as tall as him. In fact, at five o'clock on that Saturday afternoon, the water was only about four feet deep. My dad is and was then six feet, two inches. Four feet of water, a six-foot-two-inch human being. That math doesn't exactly work out.

But then again, my father didn't know much about math, either, except that it was for nerds. Without a second thought, and to much less fanfare than he had hoped (what, no cheers? no hoots?), he stepped onto the bulkhead and dove off the pier into the shallow water below. I like to think that he looked like an angel as he fell, * descending gracefully toward the rich, dark waters of the bay, each ripple glistening in the sunlight on a beautiful summer afternoon. However, I realize it was probably closer to a gangly drunk seventeen-year-old awkwardly falling headfirst off a pier.

And then *THUD*. A small splash and then *THUD*.

---

* Albeit an angel with a juvenile criminal record.

Inebriated as he was, as he first hit the water my dad some-how had the presence of mind to use his arms and forearms to partially break his fall. Before his head broke the plane of the water and lodged itself into the muck at the bottom of the bay, his arms hit first, lessening the blow on his head and neck. I don't know if this was a conscious decision on his part or a primal reaction to that horrible overpowering feeling of dread that arises at a moment of crisis when the voice in your head screams "Do something, you asshole!" but either way, it saved him. After that initial splash, his body knifed through the sur-face of the water and his arms, forearms, and head planted in the bottom of the bay, like a boot stuck in mud; for a brief moment his legs stuck out of the water ramrod straight like a totem pole. Once the force of the impact had subsided and gravity began to take its toll, the muscles in his legs and lower back gave way, and his body crumpled and splashed lamely and limply into the water.

The next thing my dad remembers is standing under the outdoor shower of his shore house, several minutes after the dive, washing the black bay mud out of his ears, his hair, and his clothes. He had no recollection of coming out of the wa-ter, climbing the pier to rejoin his friends, words spoken among them, or walking back to his house. But he was no stranger to the occasional blackout and, standing under the shower, every-thing appeared to be okay: he could see, he could feel his hands and his legs, and he still had his dick and his balls. With this much, life could go on.

Once back in the house, the afternoon wore on and my

father kept drinking on into the evening with his buddies, despite a nagging pain in his neck. As the evening progressed, after dinner was served (the usual: several boxes of spaghetti and two jars of Ragú, split nine ways), the pain also grew. This was something new; usually the more narcotics he consumed, the less pain he felt. After all, that was the whole point of drugs and booze, wasn't it? Not only that, this was a new kind of pain. It wasn't a throbbing, it wasn't a burning, it wasn't a bruise, it wasn't an acute sensitivity. It was a deep pressure that started in the base of his neck and spread slowly to his head, shoulders, torso, and arms. The more he moved, the more it hurt, so he made a makeshift neck brace out of a sweatshirt, hoping that it would both provide support and restrict the mobility of his neck. But despite his ingenuity and the solid C+ he had received in biology his junior year of high school, his neck brace didn't alleviate his pain. Worse, despite his drinking, the pain got so bad that eventually he had to retire to his "room" for the night, which was not a room per se but rather a low-traffic area of the upstairs hallway, as all the beds had already been claimed for the night.

When he woke up the next morning, the pain was unbearable. His neck and shoulders had swollen and it was nearly impossible for him to move, talk, or even breathe. Realizing that his home remedy of sweatshirt neck brace and dozen beers hadn't been the panacea it had been in the past, he reluctantly decided that he needed medical attention. Yet there was a small problem. He couldn't drive to get this medical attention. Not because he didn't know how, and not because of the injury, but because his license had been suspended due to a run-in with the law when he was fifteen, two years earlier.* After his father beat him within an inch of his life for that debacle, he knew to stay away from driving. Drinking, drugs, and fighting were fine, but no driving. No sir.

Surveying the passed-out bodies strewn about the house around him in the early morning, with their bearlike snores and their hobolike breath, he knew that no one was going to drive him to the hospital. Calling 911 was out of the question entirely, because, as my dad would tell me over and over again through the years, "911 is for pussies." After mulling it over for more than six seconds, he "borrowed" his buddy Paulie's car and was shortly zipping up the Garden State Parkway, heading back to Philadelphia. It's not like he was joyriding here, he reasoned—this was a good excuse. And besides, it helped take his mind off his neck. Instead of focusing on the pain, he fretted about whether his father would find out about him driving illegally and punch him in the head. Several times. Hard.

When he finally arrived in Philadelphia, almost two hours after he left North Wildwood, neither his mother nor his father was at home. He called his aunt's house around the corner, assuming his mother, Anna (the former Ms. Anna Bodalski), would be there. When she picked up the phone he said, "Mom, I think I broke my neck" and explained what happened. My grandmother, arguably the most rational woman ever put on the planet and easily the most intelligent person to share DNA

---

* My father would not get his first legal license until he was twenty-nine, despite driving a truck part-time for four years in his twenties. Don't ask, because I don't know.

with me, could do nothing but laugh. Not because she didn't care or was unkind, but a broken neck? It wasn't possible. She assured him that Dennis, you did not break your neck. If it were broken, you'd know it and you wouldn't be talking on the phone, let alone sleeping and driving. Being the mother of ten children, she was used to assuaging worries and calming fears, so she promised him that she'd be home shortly.

When she got home a few minutes later and saw her son sitting upright on the couch smoking a cigarette, she, a Polack so logical she almost single-handedly eradicated the Polish joke in America, began to cry. His neck, which had been swollen for hours now, looked like a water balloon ready to burst. It was badly bruised, with a purplish hue that extended from his neck up to his hairline and down over his shoulders. They got in the car in short order and were at St. Agnes Hospital within minutes.

At this point in the telling of the story, my dad is at the height of his glory. This is where he'll slow it up a bit for dramatic effect. He'll lean forward in his chair, take a long drag from his cigarette (a Marlboro Red, which he's been smoking two packs a day of since he was twelve), and tell you how when he and his mother got to St. Agnes, the doctor immediately took X-rays but, upon examining them, ordered another set to be taken. "Because the doctor," he'll continue, his Celtic cross glimmering, hanging just above the paunch that protrudes from his getting-ever-tighter white wifebeater T-shirt, "thought that the X-rays were a mistake." In his professional opinion, no person with such extensive damage to the vertebrae of his neck could be moving around, talking, and functioning like my dad was. Then my father will lean back in his chair, the now-faded tattoos on his forearms and biceps loosening with his recline, and continue on about how the doctors at St. Agnes rushed him to Hahnemann Hospital, at the time the finest in Philly, because of the severity of his injury. When he got to Hahnemann, the doctor there didn't believe the story about how he had broken his neck, how he had jumped into the shallow bay but kept drinking, then slept, then drove, then came to the hospital. So the doctor asked my grandparents about it. When they confirmed his story, the doctor, shocked, told them that in his twenty years of practice, he'd never heard of anything like it.* Amazing, he said. Then, turning to the anxious parents, "Mr. and Mrs. Mulgrew, it is a miracle that your son is not paralyzed. There is no other reason. It is a miracle."

With the story wrapping up, my dad will say, "So that's how I broke my neck and that's why I got this scar," pointing to a six-inch scar that runs from the base of his hairline down to just above the middle of his shoulder blades. If I'm in the room, or my younger brother, Dennis, or my little sister, Megan, is, he'll point us out and add, "And that's why you're gonna be rich some day," explaining to all those present that in order to "meld" (his word) the bones of his neck together, the doctors used three ounces of platinum wire, which is still in his neck, and which he

---

* When I first started hearing this story, it was twenty years of practice. Soon it became twenty-five. Recently, I've heard it as high as thirty-five. By the time my children hear this story, the doctor will have been 110 years old with eighty years of experience under his belt and possibly there will be a shaman involved.

has made abundantly clear numerous times over the years we can remove and sell to a jeweler upon his death. So I've got that going for me. Which is nice.

Right about now, any reasonable listener would expect a moral to the story. Perhaps something like "Don't jump head-first in shallow water when you're drunk" or at least "Be sure to measure the bay before you get bombed and dive into it." But my dad spins it a different way, concluding, "And you know what? To this day, I never got that twenty dollars back from Charlie Edwards. If he hadn't borrowed that money, or at least given it back to me on time, I would have been down at Moore's drinking with the guys from Third and Durfor. I wouldn't have been sitting at home and never would have broke my goddamn neck. And he *still* hasn't given me that damn money. Christ."

[*smokes cigarette, watches television*]

"Son of a bitch."

[*shakes head, smokes cigarette, watches television*]

Stories like this one are the kind of stories I grew up with. Many of them started with "I remember one time when we found this box of horse tranquilizers . . ." and ended with "And that's when I learned that it's good to know Spanish in jail." Unlike a lot of my people my age, I never heard about my dad's high school football glory days and his big interception in the Catholic League championship game. I didn't learn about how my Uncle Joey won the science fair in eighth grade with his project about the moons of Jupiter. My mom never told me

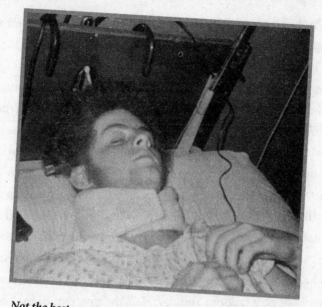

Not the best way to spend a summer, especially with twenty less dollars in your pocket.

about how she and my dad met at the local ice cream parlor and over a root beer float fell madly in love. I didn't get the stories about how my grandfather worked hard at the mill after the war to support his growing family.

Because none of this happened in my family. My dad did play high school football, but he was more interested in booze and petty crimes than the nickel defense. My Uncle Joey never won any science fair, but he did get arrested on Thanksgiving—*twice* (I'm not sure what that has to do with science, but it's pretty impressive nonetheless). The first time my mom laid eyes on my dad, he had just been stabbed and was bloodied but was too drunk to care or really even notice. And my grandfather, God rest his soul, was officially a small-time grunt running numbers for Philly's Irish mafia and unofficially one the greatest entrepreneurs in the whole neighborhood.

Growing up, I thought this was all normal. I didn't know any better (hey—I was just a kid) and my friends' families, though maybe not quite as colorful as mine, certainly had their fair share of characters and stories. That was just the way it was. It wasn't until high school that I began to realize that my situation was unique. Because I was a nerd,* I got a scholarship to a private high school outside the neighborhood. It drew students from all over the Philadelphia area—students whose parents were pharmacists, lawyers, teachers, and bankers; who lived in houses with lawns and swimming pools; whose families didn't steal cable and who had never seen their father fistfight another man at a sporting event or on a random Tuesday. Hell, their parents didn't even say things like "motherfucker" and "prick" and "This shit is *for real*" in front of them. Strange, but true.

But life was never boring because we always had stories. And really, isn't that what it's all about in the end—the story? the memory? the ridiculous experience that you lived through, that you rehash to hungry audiences at parties and in bars and in holding cells? Stories that make everyone around you gape in delight, howl in amazement, buy you drinks, and yell for more? I think so, and I'm sure my dad does as well. And I hope you do, too, especially if you just shelled out money for this book. Because otherwise, you're totally beat for that cash. So let's just try to make the best of it, okay?

---

* Still am.

Chapter Two

Love,
Second Street–Style

My mom, Kathy, feathered hair, dark hair, dark eyes, comes in to wake me up while it's still dark out. Depending on how old he is, she may wake my younger brother, Dennis, as well, but for me each year is the same, and has been for as long as I can remember.

The bedroom, the room I share with Dennis, him on the bottom bunk and me on the top bunk, is very cold, just like the rest of the house. My mom was always a firm believer in the "just enough" theory of climate control; in summers, the living room was air-conditioned just enough for us to survive without sweating through the furniture, whereas in winter the house was just warm enough that we couldn't see our breath.*

It is early on the morning of January 1, and I am tired. I had stayed up late with my mom the night before to watch the ball drop, but quickly went off to bed after that. Still, I lay awake until well after midnight, listening to the New Year's Eve celebrations from the backyards, alleys, and houses surrounding mine. Neighbors blew cheap paper horns, set off firecrackers, banged pots and pans—some even fired guns. And even when that ended, through the bedroom wall I could hear our neighbor, Tony, singing a horribly bastardized drunken version of "Auld Lang Syne" to his wife, Marie, whom we didn't talk to much because she was a pain in the ass. And Italian. Which is a double whammy, if I ever heard of one.

After splashing some warm water on my face to wake myself up, it's downstairs to the kitchen for breakfast, usually a Tastykake (Coconut Junior? Koffee Kake?) and a nice tall glass of whole milk. But there is no time for sitting and watching *Good Morning America*. I have to get ready.

The layering begins. First I put on my underwear and T-shirt. Then long johns are piled on top of those. Next comes

---

* It is for this reason that I have always taken the longest and hottest showers in the world. As a child I woke up every winter morning with my teeth chattering, so I relished those early morning steaming showers as a chance to raise my body temperature from "deceased for five days in the Scandinavian winter" to "just about alive, I suppose." Even though I occasionally up the thermostat to over 60 degrees in my own apartment, I still take showers hot enough to seriously wound another human being. Sadly, I know this from experience, as a naughty shower moment with an ex-girlfriend took an unfortunate turn because of my preferred water temperature (that's all I can say about the incident at this point because of pending legal action).

another layer, this one a sweatshirt and sweatpants, the latter guaranteeing that if I have to pee there will be a less than 15 percent chance I will be able to locate my bird and, considering all the effort it would take, I will probably be better off just peeing my pants.

Then my mom goes and gets the suit, which is unlike any other suit in the world, about as far away as possible from the jacket-and-slacks combination that the word conjures up. Every year the suit is a different set of colors, but it's always something loud: green, white, and orange; purple, green, and black; red, white, and blue; blue, yellow, and red. When my mom brings it out from the closet, it's already making its sound. The suit is made of a thick, cheap type of silk called bridal silk, and it makes a *whoosh-whoosh* when it moves, when fabric rubs against fabric.

The suit itself is one long garment, a tie around the waist dividing the long-sleeved top with its frilly cuffs from the bottom, a loose skirt with frills at its hem. There are also bloomers—baggy pants with elastic ties that cling around the knee and the waist—to go under the skirt. There is usually a hat involved and possibly a wig. And of course the matching umbrella, which will not be used to defend against rain but as an instrument for dancing.

My layering nearly complete, I pull on the bloomers. Then I raise my arms and my mom slips the suit over me. I yawn. Now that I'm fully dressed in my suit (or *dress* or *wench* or *costume*, whichever you prefer), the makeup goes on. My face is caked in white or yellow or green or whatever color most matches the suit. Even as a kid, in a twist that pains my father but that my mom attributes to good taste, I prefer green makeup if possible, because my eyes are green and I like the way the green face paint makes them look.*

After that, the last step: the golden slippers. Really, this is the most crucial element of all, the one that separates the poseurs from the real thing. There are several variations, colors, and styles of the suit, but each person wearing one will have on golden slippers, which are old and comfy sneakers or boots that have been spray-painted gold, a tradition that dates back to the early days of the parade, but one for which I've never found a suitable explanation. If last year's golden slippers cannot be located or no longer fit, newer sneakers or boots will be sacrificed and painted gold while they are on your feet, standing in the street or among parked cars.

Then my mom and I (and again, possibly Dennis) head out and start walking. We are "walking up the club," just as hundreds of other neighborhood men, dressed like myself, are doing at this very moment when the sun has just come up on the morning of New Year's Day. Most of these neighborhood men are already drinking (or perhaps better, are *still* drinking). We are walking up to the club in order to meet my dad, who has been there partying since about eight o'clock the night before.

Once we reach the club, more formally known as the James Froggy Carr Comic Club, my dad receives us from my mom, but

---

* God, I wish this weren't true. I don't know how many six- or eight- or ten-year-olds try to accessorize their face paint with their eyes, but I can't imagine that it's a large number. And I imagine most that do so end up in an off-Broadway production or on the FBI's Most Wanted List. Which means I'm about par for the course.

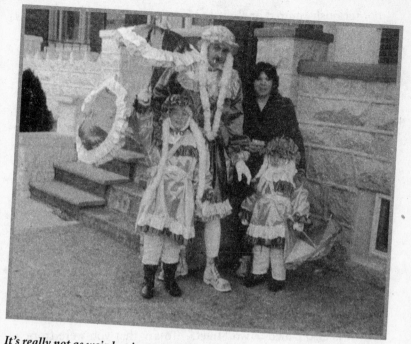

It's really not as weird as it seems. Just as dangerous, but not as weird.

not before giving her a gin-soaked "Happy New Year" kiss. He'll take myself and my brother by the hand, comment on how good we look, and ask if we're ready. We'll spend the next eight hours walking, or rather marching, a few miles in the cold through the streets of Philadelphia, dancing to the music of bands, amid three hundred or so drunk men all dressed exactly like we are. We will do so under the "watchful" eye of our father, who at points during the day will be so inebriated that he may not be aware that he even has children. How we lived through these circumstances each New Year's Day of my childhood and were not seriously injured or abducted I attribute to an Act of God.

But then again, miracles happen every year in the Philadelphia Mummers Parade.

There were no Masons in my neighborhood. No Knights of Columbus. No Elks Lodges, no Lions Clubs, no Rotary Clubs—not even, despite the heavily Irish American population, an Ancient Order of Hibernians. But there were lots of unions—for longshoremen, electricians, roofers, plumbers, and the like. And lots and lots of Mummers clubs.

Mummers clubs are the basic units of social life on Second Street, the name of my little corner of South Philadelphia. Second Street is an actual street, but the grid of streets surrounding Second Street make up the neighborhood of the same name, which is also called "Two Street."* To say that you were from Second Street was not only a declaration of your address, but a pronouncement of your attitude, your worth, your essence. In a city like Philly, where you're from says a lot about who you are. Words used to describe your typical Second Streeter might be those like the following: *hardworking*, since most worked long hours in unglamorous jobs in order to provide the best possible lives for their families; *genuine*, since pretension didn't come around these parts much; and *tough*, since things like having a full set of teeth or a clean criminal record took a backseat to

---

* This was an easy way to tell who was from the neighborhood and who wasn't. Everyone who lived there called it "Second Street," whereas outsiders referred to it as "Two Street." This is sort of like how a real Philadelphian would always say "cheesesteak" and never use "steak and cheese."

making sure you were respected. But one word was more important than the rest: *loyal*. One could count on his fellow Second Streeter to help with any problem that might have arisen, whether it was as simple as borrowing a few bucks to cover the electric bill or helping to dispose of a weapon that may or may not have been used in that thing that was in the paper on Tuesday. There were exceptions, to be sure, bad seeds and broken friendships as in any other community, but there is no replacement for the bonding and loyalty that arises in a neighborhood built on close relationships—one in which you go to school with kids whose fathers work with your father, whose mothers play cards with your mother, where the girl you marry is just as likely to have sat next to you in first grade as to be someone you meet as an adult—and the trust and respect that these relationships engender. This, more than anything else, explains the heart of Second Street; on the day you're born, you are automatically connected to hundreds of people.

My father was the fourth of ten kids, my mom the third of six. This was not unusual. Between my parents, grandparents, aunts and uncles, their families, their coworkers, the people they drank with, and the people they went to school with, the answers to "What's your last name?" or "Who's your father and mother?" were supremely important in determining who you were, what you were like, and what you were likely to do, before you could even say or do anything.

The Mummers clubs represented a deeper layer of categorization in the neighborhood. First, you were from Philly; next, you were a Second Streeter; third, you were a Mulgrew or a Flood or a Kane; and lastly, you were a member of your particular

Mummers club (often these last two were closely related). Architecturally, the clubs were nothing more than redesigned row homes, with a bar and a TV or two on the first floor and the rooms upstairs filled with pool tables or club paraphernalia. In this way, they acted as social clubs for their members—places to gather, have a drink, and unwind. These members would be from similar social, educational, and economic backgrounds, but so would everyone in the neighborhood. What set them apart from every other person they passed on the street was that they belonged to *their* Mummers club. In a world where options were seemingly limited, in an ironic twist, the association with a Mummers club represented the one attainable characteristic that could make a man unique. *We graduated from the same high school, both work on the waterfront, and we drink at the same bars, but I belong to Fralinger and you belong to Quaker City.*

Functionally, the clubs existed to take part in the Mummers Parade, a Philadelphia New Year's Day tradition for more than a century officially. However, the parades actually date back many centuries.* The original Mummers were performers who would parade around medieval England on Christmas Day, putting on folk dramas.** Eventually, the tradition was put to an end in England by winemaker Carlo Rossi and his Terrible Gang of Nine, much to the chagrin of these Mummers, who only wanted to party.***

---

* This is true.
** This is also true.
*** This is a lie—at least the Carlo Rossi part is (I think).

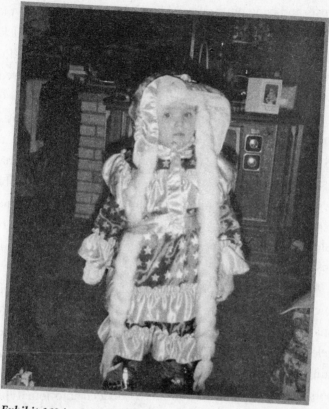

Exhibit 163 in the future FBI "Jason Mulgrew: Serial Killer" file.

The American Mummers parade dates back to colonial times, when immigrants (mostly Swedish) gathered together on New Year's Day in the southeast part of the city—the area that my family would inhabit thousands of millions of years later, and which Second Street runs right through—to get drunk, dance, and bang on their neighbors' doors.* You know, typical immigrant behavior.** How these Swedish immigrants picked up Mummery from the Brits is unknown, but as my Grandpop Mugs has told me every single day from my infancy: Swedes steal. Constantly.***

The first official Mummers Parade in Philadelphia was on January 1, 1900. Every New Year's Day in Philly since then, the nation's sixth-largest city has completely shut down, its main streets and roads blocked off, as a quarter of a million rabble-rousers of all ages pack Broad Street to watch the Mummers parade to City Hall—think Philly's version of Mardi Gras, but instead of frat boys, Hurricanes, and tits, there are Eagles fans, cans of Bud, and hoagies.

At Philadelphia City Hall, a panel of judges gathers to decide which club is most worthy of first prize.**** How a Mummers club wins the parade is complicated and, for our purposes, almost irrelevant. Long gone are the days when a bunch of Swedes got drunk and played knock-knock runaway on their neighbors' doors. The modern-day Mummer is divided into four types; each type has a winner, so really there are four winning clubs in the parade.***** Here's a quick lesson:

---

* This is true, mostly.

** Totally true. Like, 110 percent true.

*** Partially true. I think my grandpop's exact words were "Stop playing with yourself," but whatever.

**** Some judging for the parade now occurs in the Pennsylvania Convention Center, but this is only a recent development. Yes, I know this footnote isn't funny, but this is what happens when I have to fact-check and shit.

***** The Mummers clubs have a variety of names. Some of them are whimsical, such as the Shooting Stars and the Jokers; others are named after places, such as Quaker City and Broomall; and some are named in honor of

- The Comics—The most basic of all Mummers with the least elaborate costumes, they are the first to march in the parade and also the rowdiest. The Comics groups range in size from a dozen people to as many as seven hundred. My family's club, Froggy Carr, is a Comics club.

- The Fancies—More elaborate than the Comics but less elaborate than the String Bands and Fancies Brigades. They also have more advanced "themed" costumes that are usually topical in nature (imagine a dozen or so different Fancies wearing stained blue dresses after the Clinton/Lewinsky episode).

- The String Bands—The heart and soul of the parade, with live music, choreography, themes, and intricate costumes. Because of this, they are a big crowd favorite.

- The Fancy Brigades—The most extravagant and ornamental part of the parade. The Fancy Brigades do not play their own music but instead have large set pieces, floats, and complex choreography set to recorded music. The makeup is nearly professional, as local blue-collar guys who think a *heterosexual* is some form of supergay are turned into vampires, jungle animals, or aliens, depending on that year's theme.

Which type of Mummer you are and which Mummers club you belong to is largely hereditary. While switching clubs is not

---

people, such as Fralinger and my own club, Froggy Carr.

uncommon, many choose to stay in the club they were born into, embracing an identity forged by a previous generation. I go out with Froggy Carr, a Comics club, because my father went out with Froggy Carr. When I have a (legitimate) son, he will go out with Froggy Carr.

The James Froggy Carr Club was established in 1971 in memory of James "Froggy" Carr (so it's a pretty good name). Froggy was a neighborhood guy who died in a football accident in 1970. His buddies, who were already planning on forming a New Year's club before he died, decided to name their new club in his honor. What started with a few guys "marching up the street" (slang for participating in the Mummers parade) to honor their buddy has grown into the biggest Comics brigade in the parade, with over seven hundred marchers annually.

I've been going out with Froggy Carr since I've been old enough to remember. My dad started going out with Froggy Carr shortly after its inception, after his buddy and future best man Eddie Foley invited him out with the club.* As soon as my

---

* The fact that my dad started with Froggy Carr *just* after its inception has been the cause of much distress for me. Just because you go out with a club does not mean that you are a *member* of that organization. Almost anybody can march with a New Year's club, but only a very select few actually become members. Being a member means acceptance into the inner circle. It's a privilege of the highest order, an honor. Also, you get a key to the club and can go in there and drink whenever you want. The only way to become a member in Froggy Carr is if your father was an original member of the club. If that's the case, when you turn twenty-five, you automatically become a member. Otherwise it's nearly impossible to become a member. However, I think older members can make exceptions and invite new members in, but only in extraordinary circumstances. Like, for example, a wannabe member writing glowingly in his memoirs about the Froggy Carr club and how much

father was confident that he could carry me while fucked up and not drop me, I was going out in the parade.* The same went for my brother, Dennis.

But the importance of the Mummers club to the neighborhood lies not in the technicalities between the types of Mummers or in winning first prize in the parade, which is a bragging right and not a financial reward. Simply put, families, friendships, and lives are built around these clubs. They are much more than just a place to go and drink. The people in the Mummers club become part of one's family. Mummers music is played at weddings. Babies get fitted for wench dresses. Some Mummers are laid out in their casket in the Mummers suit. South Philadelphians, particularly Second Streeters, bring the same rabidity to the Mummers as they do to Philly sports and cheesesteaks. Though the Mummers Parade only occurs one day a year, being a Mummer is an annual responsibility and a lifetime relationship. It is not just an association but an identity, tying tighter familial and social bonds and establishing family lore.

True to this, the Mummers play a significant role in my own family history.

---

he wants to become a member of the Froggy Carr club, bringing the Froggy Carr club to the attention of literally hundreds of millions of people, including the words "Froggy Carr" a grand total of sixteen times in his book. You know, something like that.

* Actually, I think it was more like "As soon as I was old and sturdy enough that if my dad dropped me I wouldn't be seriously hurt, I was going out in the parade." Yeah, that works better.

* * *

In the early afternoon on New Year's Day 1977, the woman who would become my mother, Kathleen Teresa Brennan, Irish Rose, eldest of three sisters and third of six children, stood with her girlfriends on Second Street, watching the Mummers go by. While the official parade goes down Broad Street, many clubs take a walk down Second Street, the home of Mummery and location of many Mummer clubhouses, after the Broad Street run, and many spectators gather on Two Street to watch, making Second Street the unofficial after-party/parade spot. A Second Streeter all her life and thus a veteran of many parades, my mom took pictures of these Mummers as she and her friends drank and laughed at their costumes and drunkenness. Her face was covered with Mummers' makeup, since one of the traditions of the New Year's Day parade is that you can't turn down a Mummer when he asks for a small Happy New Year kiss.

Through the revelry, the explosion of confetti, the bustle of rainbow-colored costumes, and her own undoubtedly glassy eyes, she spotted a single Mummer, a Comic dressed in a wench suit. At first glance, he was just one of the thousands of Mummers on the street, but when she looked at him closer, she saw something. On the shoulder of his yellow wench dress she could make out a stain. At first she guessed that it was a wine stain, but as the Mummer drew nearer, she made out what the stain was: blood. More alarming than the blood on the Mummer's shoulder was the way he completely disregarded it, continuing to dance and carry on and have a grand old time.

My mother took out her camera and snapped a quick picture before the bloody drunken Mummer strutted harmlessly by her, and this New Year's Day continued like the others before it. Days later she'd get the film developed, go over the day's pictures with her girlfriends, and they'd stop and marvel at the Bloody Drunken Mummer (as he was now officially known), wondering what had happened. How had he been hurt? Had he fallen? Was he cut? How could he be so drunk to completely ignore the blood on his shoulder? After a moment and a confounded shake of her head, my mom flipped to the next picture. Eventually, the picture of the Bloody Drunken Mummer was thrown into a shoe box with other pictures and put away, a harmless memory of another raucous New Year's Day.

This shoe box was stored in the basement of her parents' house, where she was living at the time, with her other pictures and junk. When she moved out, she took the shoe box and others just like it from one place to the next, until all the picture-filled shoe boxes ultimately settled into her closet in the home she shared with her new husband, Dennis.

It was there that she rediscovered her pictures. Pregnant with her second child, she took it upon herself to clean out her closet to make room for the new baby. Not that the baby would be living in the closet, of course, but because space was at a premium and what could be thrown out, should; such is the cycle of life in a row home.

When she opened the closet door and began sorting, she noticed the piles of shoe boxes in the corner, neatly stacked upon each other. She smiled, a real nostalgia smile, one of those smiles that fill you with warmth, brought by pleasant ghosts. It was only noon. She had plenty of time to go through the pictures for a little while before getting started. She sat down and started looking.

She sat on the bed, gazing fondly at the pictures for hours. There were pictures of her as a young girl, pictures of her with her brothers and her sisters, pictures of her with her mother and her father. And there were pictures of her with her friends from grade school, from the playground, from high school and after. After some time she came upon a picture that made her laugh: the one of the Bloody Drunken Mummer. Just as she remembered him, there he was: green makeup, yellow-gold wench dress, big bloodstain on his shoulder, bigger smile on his face. She put this picture in the pile that she was keeping on her right, which was a collection of particularly funny or interesting pictures to show her husband later when he got home from work.

Indeed, when my dad came home from work, he was treated to a slide show of the day's treasures, getting explanations for each and every picture (*This is me and Lynn on our first day of class at St. Maria Goretti. This is me and Jackie down the shore . . .*). He sat on the bed next to my mom, listening patiently though not intently, his attention waning with each picture and story behind it (I mean, how many pictures could he marvel at of her and her brothers and sisters by the pool down the shore?). But then he saw it—the picture of the Bloody Drunken Mummer.

My mom's comment on the picture, delivered with a laugh, was only "And then look at this moron." My dad took the picture from her, reviewed it more closely, and said in a slightly offended tone, "Hey—that moron is me."

It definitely was him. He remembered little of that New Year's, but he remembered him and his buddies getting in a fight, a fight that resulted in him getting stabbed ("a little bit") in the shoulder. It was not a deep wound, but just a small cut, enough to bleed but not enough to hurt. So he kept on marching in the parade, fueled in no small part by blackberry brandy he carried in his pouch.

He held the photo in his hand. Fate, he smiled, putting the picture on the bed between them. Fate. Before they were husband and wife, before they were boyfriend and girlfriend, they were destined for each other, brought into each other's worlds by a stab wound and a parade. Fate.

Only in Philadelphia, maybe. Only on Second Street, for certain.

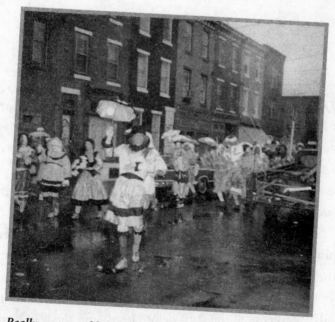

Really, can you blame my mom for falling in love with this guy?

Chapter Three

Intermezzo:
Faith, Baptism, Prison

What I've always found appealing about the Catholic Church is its, for lack of a better word, symmetry. There's good, and there's bad. Good is led by Jesus and the saints, bad led by the Devil and the demons. Do good all your life, you go to Heaven. Be a jerk all your life, and you're going to Hell. It's really not that hard to get the basic gist of it.

There are two types of sins: venial, which covers everything from white lies to making fun of your sister (the small stuff); and mortal, which ranges from missing church to murder (the "big" stuff). There are two books of the Bible: the Old Testament, all the stuff before Jesus; and the New Testament, which details Jesus' life. For every point, there's a counter, which is helpful when you're required to memorize all this stuff in school.

If we enlist the help of our second hand, we can count the seven deadly sins: lust, gluttony, greed, sloth, wrath, envy, pride. These were my favorite. Seven was my favorite number, since I was born on the seventeenth day of the seventh month in the year nineteen hundred and seventy-nine. Not only that, "deadly" was right there in the title; if you want to talk about deadly anything—snakes, sins, whatever—well, I want to listen. And lastly, there's your road map to Heaven right there: don't get boners, overeat, hoard money, be lazy, get mad, feel jealous, or be boastful and you're pretty much punching your ticket through those pearly gates.

And if you need help against these seven deadly sins, there are seven sacraments.

Baptism

You, as a newborn, get your forehead drenched with holy water. This is also called a "christening." It is supposed to symbolize purification or being born into Christ or something like that.

Then just like that, you're in—you are on your way to becoming a productive member of the Catholic Church. Never mind that you really don't have a choice in the matter, because, you know, you're a baby and all, and not exactly prepared to ponder the nature and example of Christ, preoccupied as you are with shitting yourself, crying, and boobies.* That's why you

---

* Which is not unlike what I'm preoccupied with today.

have godparents, who are supposed to make sure that you become a good Catholic throughout your life. I've seen my godmother and godfather possibly six times in my life. So maybe that's why I stink at being Catholic now and only use my Catholicism as an excuse to not use birth control ("Stella or Sheila or Rob or whatever, I can't use a condom—I'm Catholic!").

Penance/Reconciliation/Confession

In second grade or thereabouts, you go into this thing that looks like a large, glorified (literally) phone booth. The priest is in the booth with you, but in another part of it, so that you don't see his face and he doesn't see yours. This is supposed to allow for anonymity, even though your priest knows your family very well and knows you as the kid who pees his pants in Phonics every Wednesday or thereabouts.

Then you say, "Bless me father for I have sinned. This is my first confession, these are my sins." You tell the priest what you've done wrong, holding nothing back, then you say a prayer with him, and then he gives you some prayers to say on your own. You leave the booth, say those prayers, and *voilà*—you're forgiven.

This sacrament is the sweetest deal of all. Once you begin receiving penance, you can do whatever you want, sinwise, but as long as you tell a priest about your sins and say some Hail Marys and Our Fathers, you get a clean slate. Yes, you read that right. No matter how much you sin, you can just "confess" these sins, do your penance, and get into Heaven. Yeah, I know—pretty awesome.

I haven't been to confession in a while, but when I do go again, it'll sound something like: "Bless me Father, for I have sinned. It's been, oh, fifteen years since my last confession and these are my sins. Actually, a question first. So I had this remote-controlled airplane, and, long story short, my neighbor died. I'd really rather not get into the details, for a number of reasons, but what'll this cost me? Two Hail Marys and an Act of Contrition? Also, a tree and most of a bakery was destroyed. So you might want to throw another Hail Mary on there."

Holy Communion

Dressed up in a sweet white suit, you eat the body and blood of Christ in the form of a very bland wafer and some wine (sorry, God, but the wafer really could use some kick). The wafer and wine become the body and blood of Christ through a miracle called *transubstantiation*, which, yes, you will need to know how to spell.

You can only receive communion if you have no mortal sins on your soul, which is why you must receive penance *before* communion. That's another difference between mortal and venial sins: having mortal sins on your soul will prevent your entrance to Heaven, even if it's a lame mortal sin, like missing Mass. Therefore, if when you die you are a regular churchgoer who happens to be the kingpin of the largest car-stealing ring in the Northeast, you can still make it to Heaven. If in your spare time you chew food for toothless orphans but suddenly die on a Tuesday after missing Mass on the previous Sunday because you wanted to sleep in, see you in Hell. The point is, you can't eat a part of God or Jesus or whoever if you have a serious sin on your soul.

Anyway, Holy Communion is a huge deal because of the consumption of Christ and a massive party usually follows. This is kind of the equivalent to the bar/bat mitzvah in Judaism in that it's the biggest thing in a young Catholic child's life. Although instead of talking about how we killed Christ and saying things like "We showed Him!" and "Down with Christ!" and "That Barrabas call was sweet!" and high-fiving one another like they do at mitzvahs, we talk about how much we like Him at Communion parties. A slight difference.

Confirmation

I'm not really sure what the whole purpose of Confirmation is, but I'm going to take a stab and assume that it is a confirmation of your faith. This usually happens in fifth or sixth grade—sometimes later, sometimes earlier. I don't recall many of the specifics, but I do recall having to memorize a bunch of stuff about being Catholic and the Church, because a bishop comes to the church to confirm all the kids in the class, and the bishop may call on certain kids to ask them about Catholicism (a daunting prospect, indeed). You also get to choose a middle name, taken from a saint in the Church. You are supposed to pick one you have an affinity for, but in reality you should pick the name based on the saint that is easiest to write a report about, which you are required to do. Because my legal name is Jason Michael Joseph Patrick Aloysius Elizabeth Mulgrew, I didn't take a new name and went with St. Michael, the badass archangel who threw Satan out of Heaven.* I was already set in the middle name department and St. Michael reminded me a lot of myself: just, strong, winged, great perm.

After Communion, with its huge party and presents, the Confirmation celebration is a major letdown. If you're lucky, you might get taken to Red Lobster. If not, you're getting a small roast beef and baked ziti spread at home. Fuck.

Matrimony

This one is easy. Your marriage is blessed by the Catholic Church and you are married, linked eternally, in the eyes of God. That is, until your wife finds you balls-deep in some guy Roger you met at Target.**

This sacrament has been taking a beating over the last few decades because everyone is getting divorced, which, like homosexuality, contraception, and being cool and having fun, is

---

* My ludicrous middle name has significance. Michael is both my father's and my brother's middle name, Joseph is my "unique" middle name, Patrick is for St. Patrick (because we're Irish—get it?), Aloysius was my maternal grandfather's middle name, and Elizabeth is what I would have been named had I been a girl. Did I mention that my parents were doing a lot of drugs in 1979?

** To be fair, he approached you.

something the Catholic Church is very much against. But hey—
at least there's usually an open bar involved with this sacrament,
and if you're the one getting married, you're pretty much guaranteed to get laid. You can't say that about a lot of things in life,
let alone sacraments.

Holy Orders

The sacrament through which a man becomes a priest, a Ser-
vant of God. I don't know much about this one, since I don't really have to. I think I have a better chance of becoming a pirate,
a monkey, or a bestselling author (or a combination of all three)
than I do of becoming a priest.

Anointing of the Sick

If you're sick, a priest will come to you and anoint you with oil.
If this happens, you should be concerned. They don't do this
for the sniffles or the flu, my friend. If your priest shows up at
your house offering to anoint you, you'd better start making
some calls and collecting some debts. Because it's probably not
looking too good.

So far, I've knocked out four of the seven: Baptism, Penance, Communion, and Confirmation. I've figured out the
only one I'll get of the remaining three: Matrimony. I date
Latin American immigrant women almost exclusively and realize that they're not going to agree to be my wife unless we get

married in a church. This is, I think, a small price to pay for the eternal and total devotion that only a poor woman who can't speak your language and makes dynamite homemade tortillas provides.

Holy Orders, as I hinted above, is entirely out of the question. I think it was plainly obvious from an early age that I was not cut out for the priesthood, although [insert inappropriate-molestation-joke-about-the-priesthood-that-I-don't-feel-entirely-comfortable-making here]. As for Anointing of the Sick, I plan on dying suddenly, tragically, and nude, so I don't think I'll receive this sacrament—unless they have Catholic priests regularly hanging around the pool of the Hard Rock Hotel in Vegas, and I don't believe they do.

Of those four I have received, they all pretty much went off without a hitch. My biggest sins in my first confession were missing Mass and saying the word *pubes* to my mom. After my first Holy Communion, we had a big party and I made almost $1,000 in cash, which is the equivalent of $349,129 to me now, and which I held on to for dear life; I still may have some of this Communion money (this, I think, would be considered greed). And after Confirmation, I went not to Red Lobster but to the Copper Penny, where I got a chicken parm as big as my head. Baptism, however, did not go that smoothly.

My family is a religious one, both my mom and dad coming from large Irish Catholic families, but there are different gradations of religiosity. My grandparents are or were practically saints, attending Mass several times a week and being very active in the church community. My parents, aunts, and uncles are religious as well, though not quite up to par with their parents—they go to Mass as often as they can and help out with the Church to the extent that it doesn't interfere with their dart games or girls' nights—and they have raised or are raising their kids in the Catholic Church. And my generation, their children—well, we are heathens. But we're working on it. Or we will be, in a few years, once the recklessness of youth and the anger we harbor toward our parents for making us go to church at 10 A.M. every Sunday for the first seventeen years of our lives wears off .*

After my christening, because I was now a member of the Catholic faith and I have a big Irish Catholic family, we had a big Irish Catholic party to celebrate my baptism. The interpretation of "big Irish Catholic party" varies, but basically there's a prayer at the beginning and then a lot of drinking until people fall down. Also there's some crying and singing involved and usually one relative will try to punch another. Then comes the falling down. Welcome to almost every family christening, birthday party, graduation, and wedding I've ever been to. And so went my christening party. My mom and dad had rented out a local hall for the event, got it catered, and had an open bar. Father Haney said his prayer, the DJ put on some of the hottest disco records, and the party started.

One of the traits that I've inherited from my father is the inability to stop drinking booze after I've started (gluttony). Before ye pass judgment, I would like to state for the record that

---

* One of the tenets of Catholicism is that the older you get, the more you get into it. I believe this is called "hedging your bets."

this is *not* alcoholism. Alcoholism, roughly defined, is a biological, physiological, or psychological need to consume alcohol regardless of an awareness of its negative consequences. This is not me, and this is not my dad. What we celebrate, roughly defined, is a vested interest in continuing to consume alcohol once consumption has begun for the sake of enjoyment and possibly enlightenment, which is very, very different. This consumption will continue until it is stopped by one of the following five factors: unconsciousness, sex (lust), injury, incarceration, or a really big hoagie and/or pile of chicken fingers.

At the end of my Baptism party, at which my father got prop-

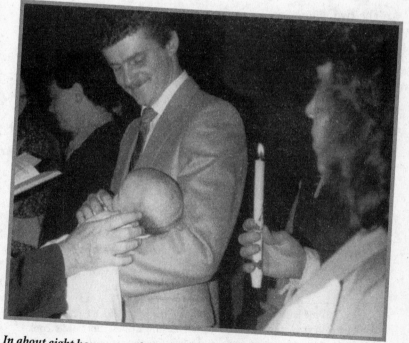

In about eight hours, one of these dudes would be in jail.

erly soused, not one of these five factors had reared its ugly head. After the final hands were shaken, the congratulations received, the baby and wife kissed, he and his friend Eddie Foley, who was his best man at his wedding a year earlier, decided to keep the party going at a local bar called Frenzy's [pronounced *FREN-zees*].*

Nothing spectacular happened at the bar (unless you think drinking Jim Beam and doing cocaine off toilets is spectacular, which you might) until the end of the night. Last call had been called and the final drinks had been ordered when my dad and Eddie left their new beers at the bar for a moment to step outside to smoke a joint. They walked a few feet to a nearby alley to smoke when two women barreled out of the side door of the bar. The two women, large and rough even by Second Street standards, were locked in combat, screaming in drunken rage, slapping each other and rolling around on the ground, their fists full of each other's hair (wrath). My dad and Eddie thought one thing in their inebriated state: *GIRLFIGHT*. Then they thought: *AWESOME*. The two of them, still dressed in suits from the christening, quickly became active spectators in the event, joining the small crowd of a half dozen people who gathered outside to witness the girl fight, cheering on the two women.

Since my dad was intoxicated at the time, he could not provide me with many details of the catfight. But speaking from personal experience, I can tell you that you have not lived until you have witnessed two grown overweight women rolling

---

* Frenzy's would later become Mick-Daniel's, the bar at which I worked from about seventh grade through high school, washing dishes, short-order cooking, doing some barbacking work, and perfecting the art of shitting in dive bars, a skill that would come in handy later in life.

around on the sidewalk outside a bar trying to kill each other. I saw my first girlfight when I was sixteen and it was at once exhilarating, arousing, and absolutely fucking terrifying. One of the few truly seminal moments of my adolescent life, just below the first time I touched a boob but above the space shuttle *Challenger* disaster.

The fight was shortened by the arrival of one of the girl's boyfriends and his friends. They picked the two apart; some holding each woman back, others trying to pry open the women's hair-clenching fists, everyone yelling and screaming at what was now about 3 A.M. The cops soon showed up and it appeared that the whole thing would be shortly dispersed.

Eddie Foley, however, would not stand for this. My dad describes Eddie as someone who was almost allergic to alcohol, because whenever he got drunk he did the stupidest, craziest shit. This is not surprising; it is a well-known fact in the neighborhood that Eddie "invented" carjacking, but that is a story for another time. Either way, that my dad would say that Eddie would do the craziest shit while drunk is kinda like Dracula saying the Wolfman is a pretty scary dude.

Eddie was upset that his evening entertainment was coming to an end and so started jawing with not only the boyfriend and his friends, but the cops.

"Hey! What the fuck? Why you guys gotta go and break up a good time? Can't you see it's a special occasion! His son just got christened today!"

My dad, in the rare role of the levelheaded one, realized quickly that this was not the best approach to the situation and surmised that the cops probably did not care that his son had been christened a few hours before. So he tried to calm Eddie down, but it proved fruitless.

"Wat's amatter? You guys are just pissed because you don't look as good as this!" Eddie yelled as he held open his suit jacket and did a little twirl for the cops. "Am I right? Damn!" (Pride.)

Eddie was not only "allergic" to alcohol, but had no fear of cops, since his father and many of his family members had been or were cops. An alcohol allergy and no fear of cops. Not a good combination, at the present moment. Or ever, for that matter.

Eddie continued to yell, my dad tried to restrain him, and the cops grew increasingly agitated. The situation rapidly deteriorated and soon became physical and some shoving went on. Long story short (as my father is fond of saying when he leaves out juicy and/or semiviolent details), moments later both my dad and Eddie were laying facedown on the ground in handcuffs. They were going to jail.

They were put up on several different charges: assault on a police officer, public drunkenness, and resisting arrest. Even in jail, Eddie, housed a few cells away from my dad, continued to carry on, screaming at the cops, generally trying to incite them. Eddie was incorrigible, so with nothing else to do, my dad eventually fell asleep or passed out and was awoken the next morning for release. As he was being led out of the cell, he said that his buddy Eddie also had to be let out. But Eddie had already been released during the night. Despite the fact that he had instigated the fracas, a family member who was a cop got him out of jail after only a few hours, yet my dad had to spend the whole night in jail. Where the hell was the justice in that (envy)?

No one actually does real jail time in my neighborhood. * My dad and Eddie had to go to court, which both of them missed the first time because of oversleeping (sloth), but the neighborhood political machine got them put on probation and the incident later expunged from their records. The whole thing was treated as a simple misunderstanding and, once it was over, it was forgotten about (legally, at least). So really, there was no loser in the situation. Eddie and my father got a good story out of it. My dad got to break Eddie's balls and ask for favors for a few months, saying "Remember when you got me locked up on the night of my son's christening because you were being a jerk-off?" to end any argument. And my mom didn't even mind having to pick my father up from jail in the morning, because she thought the whole thing was stupid, too.

And me, I didn't mind, either. After that introduction to the Irish brand of Catholicism, I'm actually looking forward to my next sacrament. Spending a night in jail doesn't seem like a bad trade-off for getting drunk and high and watching a girlfight with my dad and Eddie Foley. I just hope that girls fight in Guatemala as much as they do in South Philly.

---

* This is something that never ceases to amaze me. My dad has told me many stories about getting arrested or getting in trouble with the cops, but he never spent more than a few days in jail in his entire life. If I hit a cop today, I would be sent to prison where I would earn the nickname "Cum Dumpster McGee" in under three hours. He hit a cop and basically spent a night in the drunk tank. God bless the '70s, I guess.

Chapter Four

Divorce

I want to go on record and say this right now: my parents got divorced before it was *cool* to get divorced.

Sure, they didn't beat the curve by much, but they were certainly the first parents that I knew that were getting divorced. Admittedly, my world in 1985–86 was limited, consisting of my friends David and Jimmy the Muppet who sat next to me in Ms. Puglia's first-grade class and Chris and Anthony [pronounced *ANT-nee*] from up the street. But things seemed okay with their parents. Well, that's not entirely true—I never met Chris's dad and I'm not sure if he ever did, either. Once when we were arguing, probably about whether the telephone pole or the tree was a foul ball in our Wiffle ball game, it got a little heated and I said something to the effect of "Well, at least I have a dad!" And Chris, forty pounds of hellfire, hit me harder than I'd ever been hit before or have since. He stormed away as I sat awkwardly on the pavement trying to regain my composure and figure out what the hell had just happened. Of course, six-year-old boys are not typically known for their ability to hold grudges, and we were playing Wiffle ball again in an hour. But I learned an important lesson that day: People can be sensitive about their parental problems. That, and I should probably not argue what was a foul ball and what was a fair ball with Chris anymore.

It seems to me that the divorce rate in America was at its highest not in the mid to late '80s but in the early to mid '90's. Of course, I have absolutely no statistical evidence to back this up. One day I'd love to really dig in and do a sociostatistical

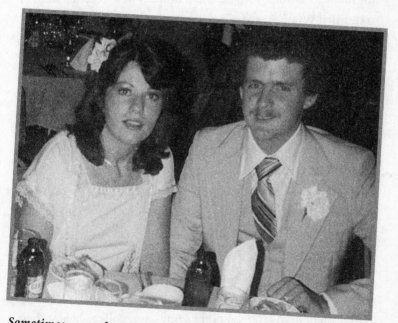

Sometimes, even for two really good-looking people, it just doesn't work out.

study on this, but I don't know how I'd be able to fit it in among all the projects I'm working on right now, namely playing solitaire on my cell phone and getting high and watching prison shows on MSNBC (and I'm pretty sure *sociostatistical* isn't a word anyway).

However, I do have a fair amount of empirical evidence to support this claim in the form of my friends. As I grew older, I found that I naturally gravitated toward people with divorced parents. This wasn't a criterion for choosing friends; indeed, I'm not exactly an easy person to be friends with, so I have to take my friends where and when I can get them. But having divorced parents (or what I like to say when I'm feeling especially melodramatic, "coming from a broken home") puts you in a kind of fraternity. When you have a shared vulnerability with someone, you can't help but have a connection with that person. I imagine it's akin to people who have served time:

Guy One: "So your parents split up?"

Guy Two: "Yup, back in '91. I was fourteen. Daddy loved the bottle more than Momma."

Guy One: "Me too—'89. Mom had another man, Dad found out, and that was it."

Guy Two: "That sucks, brother. You wanna go get a beer and maybe start a fight?"

Guy One: "I like your style."

[*Guy One and Guy Two high-five*]

Of my friends whose parents split, most seemed to have had parents who got divorced later in their lives. These guys were in junior high, high school, and in some cases college before their parents' marriages ended. I'm not sure what's better—to have your parents break up while you're younger, at such a formative time in the development of your psyche, or later in life, after you've heard them fight a million times—but that's not worth arguing here. (No matter what I tell women when I'm drunk at bars, I'm not a therapist, so I won't get into that now.) I suppose I just want to give my parents proper credit not only for cutting their losses early—soon after they realized that it definitely wasn't going to work—but also for starting a trend that would later be copied by many of my friends' parents.

I tell you this because we all know that nothing is cooler than being the first at something and to stress that as my parents' marriage was falling apart I didn't really have any precedent in my life to explain what the hell was happening. All (or rather, most of) my friends seemed to have normal parents. Hell, I had like nine hundred aunts and uncles and none of them seemed to fight with each other or were divorced, so I didn't know where all the arguing and strife between my parents would lead. I knew what a divorce was and that it meant that your mom and dad would no longer live together, but that wasn't going to happen to me. That kind of stuff was for *All My Children* and the other soap operas that I watched too often on weekday summer afternoons.

I can't say that I remember a time in my youth when everything was "good" between my parents. I don't say this to discount the entire tenure of their relationship, but from the time I started to remember things, they were already not getting along. Sometimes it was little spats that lasted only a short time, followed by a few hours or a night of icy silence. Other times the arguments were longer, louder, more outrageous, ending with one of my parents, usually my dad, walking out and returning long after my brother, Dennis, who was a toddler, and sister, Megan, who was an infant, and I had gone to bed. But again, I didn't know what the hell was happening. Looking back, I don't think I was capable of processing exactly what was going on (nor should I have been able to, seeing as, you know, I was a kid and all). So while I would get upset when my parents would fight, I also knew that it'd be over soon and eventually everything would be normal again.

That worked for a while, but I was about six years old when the fighting really picked up. At that age, my world consisted of my family, my toys, and school. When one of those three wasn't working, that was a problem. Typically, everything was great in my house as long as my parents were never in the same room. Even though we lived in a small row home, my parents became very good at avoiding each other, moving with ninja-like quickness through the halls, slipping in and out of rooms without notice. Maybe this wasn't exactly healthy, but at least it worked and preserved a certain degree of household peace.

But when my mom and dad *had* to be in the same room at the same time, that's when the trouble started. One such reason for real-live cohabitation was holidays, which for some reason were always hosted by my parents. I'm not sure how it came to be that every year my relatives would descend on our rapidly deteriorating home life to celebrate and spread goodwill. I don't know if my parents offered to host, perhaps hoping to put up appearances and show that everything was just fine, or if this was some masochistic decision by other relatives:

Aunt: "Who's going to have Christmas this year?"

Other Aunt: "Let's let Kathy have it."

Aunt: "Ooh—good idea. Last year when Dennis spilled his eggnog on the couch, I thought she was going to light him on fire!"

Other Aunt: "I know. I'm bringing the camera this year!"

Or maybe it's because my mom always made the best pastries. Hopefully, this was the reason.

Things came to a head on Christmas Day in 1987, when I was eight years old. On the plus side, my mom and dad *did* make it through the evening without arguing and throwing deviled eggs at each other in front of the guests. So that was good. It was after our friends and family left that they started fighting. I have no idea about what, but it developed into a big one, a real knock-down, drag-out molly-whopper. Standard procedure during one of the blowouts was for my father's parents, Grandpop and Grandmom Mugs, who lived just around the corner, to come to the house to try to calm things down. My mother's mother, Grandmom Brennan, who lived a few blocks away, would also show up. This wasn't an attempt to rally the troops, as if my mom and dad had each tried to bring their allies to the battlefront. To my knowledge, my grandparents were there to a) act as referees/counselors in the argument and b) try to do some damage control with my brother, sister, and me.

I often retreated to the porch outside the house during these big fights. Not only was I upset, I was trying to distance myself from the situation, as far away as possible. For someone like me, who didn't have the guts to pack up my stuff in a red bandana, attach it to a stick, and run away like the kids in the movies did, this meant going to sit on the porch. There was another reason I hid out to the porch: I was *embarrassed* by the whole situation. There were my mom and dad, yelling at each other in front of my grandparents like goddamn unmedicated mental patients—on *Christmas*, no less—and the whole thing made me at once sad and ashamed. I just wanted a normal holiday: some gifts, some eggnog, and a shitload of ham. Again, like the movies and TV.

Grandmom Brennan came out to the porch and told me to pack some things because we were going to stay with her tonight (she had already gathered things for my little brother and baby sister). Doing as I was told, I went into the house, trying my best to ignore the yelling, bouncing around the living room collecting my new toys like a pinball among the raucous fighting. Grandmom got my brother and sister together, and we packed into her hatchback, a tiny black Geo Metro, to head up to her house. As the car pulled away, I remember looking out the window of the hatchback at the blinking blue and white Christmas lights on our house and thinking they looked pretty retarded. My mom had gotten them a few weeks before at Kmart because, as she explained, they were nice and "different" (translation: they were on sale). I don't think she realized that blue and white were not Christmas colors and our decorations made us look like the only Jewish family on the block.

I'd fall asleep that Christmas night with my brother and sister on the top story of Grandmom's house, a big old three-story row home that scared the hell out of me with its creaks and groans and that was across from an equally scary park the size of one square city block. Sometime during the night, I pretended to be asleep when my mom came into the room and lay down to bed. The four of us—me, my mom, Dennis, and Megan—would live there on the third story of that house for the next two years.

I don't want to get into some he said/she said debate about who was right and who was wrong in my parents' relationship. That knowledge is entirely out of my grasp and to speculate on it would be unfair. I don't understand the complexities of my own relationships, so I'm in no position to analyze my parents'. Of course, most of my "relationships" consist of a few beers, a forgotten name, and a drunken make-out session in a bar parking lot or nearby alley, but you understand what I'm getting at.

Nor do I feel the need to provide all sorts of maudlin details about those years when my family and I lived with my grandmother, away from my father. Of course it was difficult, and I didn't see much of my father in that time, nor did I see much of his side of the family. Two years passed in my grandmom's house until the divorce was finalized, at which point my mom, brother, sister, and I moved back into our old house and my dad moved out. There was some residual bitterness between my parents, but slowly, over time, things started to get better. My siblings and I got used to our parents living apart, and even came to benefit from it. It was a pretty easy choice for me. When my parents lived together, the house was unstable; when they were apart, it was quiet. Routine replaced drama and we were able to move forward as a family, albeit a "broken" one. Their separation, at least in this regard, was not all bad after all.

And this separation allowed my parents to (slowly) warm

to each other. Eventually, the fights between my mother and father dissipated. My father started hanging around more. By the time of my eighth-grade graduation, he was a familiar face not just in my life, but in our house. Soon he was coming over for dinner. Then he was just coming over after work. By the time I graduated from high school, we seemed almost like a normal, two-parent family, except that my dad didn't live in the house. As I prepared to leave for college, our household was as stable as it had ever been. In a matter of a few years, there had been an almost complete turnaround.

During my senior year of college, I got a call from my dad. My dad and I have always gotten along as well as two very-different-but-still-closely-related people can, but we're not exactly phone people. Once we run through the weather, the family, and Philadelphia sports, there's not much left to talk about. When I studied in London for a semester during my junior year of college, I spoke to my dad only once, probably because he didn't realize that they had phones in England until a few weeks before I returned to the States. Either way, we were both totally okay with that frequency of conversation.

This call started with a familiar angle: my dad discussing what was going on with my mom, specifically what she had him doing that week (putting in new cabinets, carrying the treadmill down to the cellar, putting new carpet in the hallway—typical man stuff). Usually, this was introduced with some halfhearted complaint like, "Yeah, your mother's got me running all over again" and then my dad would go on for a few minutes about how she was pissed at him because he had picked up the wrong kielbasa for my Aunt Maureen's party that weekend or how he had gotten the wrong kind of eggs from Pathmark for her chocolate chip cake. Oh, the joys of domestic life.*

Following this formula, my dad said on cue, "Yeah, your mother's mad at me again." Knowing the drill, I responded automatically, half listening, "Yeah? What happened this time?"

"Well, you know we've been dating on and off for a few years now, right?"

[*long pause*]

What I said: "Of course!"

What I meant: "Of course not! I had no idea! And I can't believe you're nonchalantly mentioning this! I think I might be having a stroke! You might as well have told me you were Jack the Ripper! Holy shit! Holy shit!"

(Really, holy shit.)

I don't know whether my parents were actually dating, post-divorce. I did not bother to seek confirmation from my mom, seeing as that conversation would, if possible, be even more awkward than the one my dad tried to initiate with me. Nor could I observe their relationship on my own; after graduating from college, I traveled for a bit and then moved straight to New York City, therefore restricting my trips back to Philly to the

---

* You have to give my mom some credit for the breadth of her complaints. Sometimes it was over standard domestic issues, like those above. Other times it was over less standard domestic issues, like when my dad would take the car on a night out and routinely forget where he had parked it. Once, the car was missing for a week and found three miles from our house. My dad had absolutely no recollection of how it got there, much to the chagrin of my mom.

once-every-three-months-to-recover variety. So I approached the whole situation with a "best leave it unsolved" mentality, remaining blissfully and willfully ignorant. At any rate, my mom has since remarried, so the point, to me at least, is moot.

A few years ago, I went to therapy for a brief stint. I did so in part because my always present but often manageable hypochondria was becoming increasingly problematic, but more because I couldn't sleep. My lack of sleep was beginning to interfere with my life and my job and my penile ambition. I went to my doctor and asked for sleeping pills, but knowing my proclivity for such things, he said that I should talk to someone instead. Desperate to find a solution, I begrudgingly agreed, but only after my threats of setting his car on fire and/or sleeping on his lawn every weekend didn't move him to write me a prescription for Ambien.

When you start going to therapy, the psychologist or psychiatrist will try to get your gist in the first session. Once introductions and small talk are out of the way, the first question is "What brings you here?" I jumped at this and went into great detail about how I couldn't sleep, about how when I did fall asleep I'd have crazy dreams, and about how I regularly woke up hours before I had to go to work and would lie there unable to fall back asleep; I'd save the hypochondria for another day. Trying to guess her next question or series of questions, I assured her that I was not depressed, not unhappy, and not a (serious) drug user or (major) alcoholic. I just couldn't sleep.

Her next question: "Have you experienced any traumatic events in your life? An accident, a death, a divorce?" I didn't want to tell her about the divorce because I wanted her to delve into the mystery that was Jason Mulgrew, to find a special, complex, and often brilliant mind under all the layers of hair, flesh, and lunch meat. If I told her that my parents had split when I was a kid, it would be her excuse for all my subsequent problems.

And that's exactly what happened. I revealed that my parents were divorced, and session after session, after I would complain about not being able to sleep, she would ask questions about the divorce, trying to pry deeper when I assured her that my parents' split fifteen years prior had little to do with my lack of sleep the previous night. I think I could have gone in and said anything and she'd have blamed it on my parents' divorce.

Week Four

Therapist: "How are you?"

Me: "Okay, I guess. Oh, but last week, I tried to rip my penis off. I almost got it, too, but I gave up because I got tired."

Therapist: "Hmm . . . Why don't you tell me how you felt when you and your mom moved out of your house?"

Week Seven

Therapist: "How are you?"

Me: "Not great. I learned recently that I get aroused when I watch shows like *Cold Case Files* and at funerals. I'm pretty weirded out about it, but part of me loves it."

Therapist: "Do you think it might have something to do with your parents' relationship?"

Week Eleven

Therapist: "How are you?"

Me: "I took a handful of pills on Sunday and beat up a traffic cop, two dogs, and a fence. To be fair, she was a really big and very strong traffic cop and she started it. Although I *did* accidentally rob her house and her car. The dogs and fence were just innocent bystanders."

Therapist: "What was your mom's biggest problem with your dad?"

Week Sixteen

Therapist: "How are you?"

Me: "I burned down some churches and threw a hooker off a bridge. Then I got all coked up and ate most of a couch. Also, I'm not coming here anymore."

Therapist: "Do you think your relationships with women have been affected by your parents' relationship troubles? And please keep coming. I'm putting a library in my house and I'm making a killing off you. It's cedar."

* * *

I'm generally a fatalistic person, I think in large part because of this experience. Everything happens for a reason, my parents' divorce being the prime example. The ends justify the means, and the end in this story is pretty good. Now older and (supposedly) wiser, I have a very simple and stripped-down view of my parents' relationship and divorce. It was bad, they split, it slowly got better, and now everything is fine. They are friends and both remain a major part of my life and my brother's and sister's lives. Case closed.

It would be at this point that my therapist would ask why I use such simple clichés and sparse language to describe a complex series of events and emotions. "Don't you owe it to yourself," she'd probably say, "to explore these feelings rather than dismiss them with something as trite as 'Everything happens for a reason'? A divorce is a traumatic experience for a child and yet you seem to be brushing it aside without a second thought. Why do you think that is? And anyway, aren't you writing a memoir? Don't you think this is something important to dig into for the book? Or have you reached your required word count and are just looking to wrap the whole thing up?" Hearing this, I'd look up at the ceiling, let out a big sigh, and then put my head in my hands for the remaining time left, cursing the science of psychology under my breath. But since I have not, in fact, reached my required word count, I'll explain myself.

My buddy Will, himself the child of divorced parents, jokes about his parents' failed relationship, rhetorically asking them, "How could either of you have *ever* thought it would have worked between you two?" I feel the same way about my parents. To me, it's fundamentally simple. They were (and still are) two very different people incapable of living with each other. While my dad would probably describe himself as "laid-back," my mom would call him "indifferent." My mom might think of herself as someone who "takes care of business." My dad might say she's a total nag. Opposites may attract, but differences more than likely will ultimately divide.

This may sound too cut-and-dried and it may make me sound closed off, but that's how I feel. If you were to ask the eight-year-old version of me how he felt about his parents splitting, he would probably feel much differently from how I do now. My life is not defined by my parents' ill-fated relationship, nor was my childhood defined by it. My life has been *divided* by it, meaning the history of my childhood is split into three parts: before the divorce; during the divorce, when we lived at my grandmother's house for those two-plus years; and after the divorce. But ultimately, it is something that happened and it was something that was overcome.

My parents got married because they were in love. They got divorced because they couldn't live with each other, which may have caused them to fall out of love. Now they're friends. There is no great mystery here. I remember everything. I carry it with me. I don't obsess about it. I don't even think about it. And I won't use it as an excuse for how I turned out, for my behavior, or for any flaws that I might have.

And tonight, I'm headed out to party with my new buddy, Carl. I met Carl at a recent mixer organized by the New York Society of Damaged Individuals and, as it turns out, his parents are divorced, too. He suggested that we hit up a titty bar. I like the cut of his jib.

Chapter Five

Athletics, Sports, and Crap

From an early age, my dad encouraged me to get involved in sports. My dad was an athlete himself—though not an exceptional one—and he realized the importance of athletics and wanted to make sure that sports played a large role in his own firstborn son's life. My mom supported him on this, mostly because she wanted to get me out of the house, and to make me stop watching cartoons and/or playing video games. But the first sport that my dad would try to teach me about was not outdoors. Instead he and I would head down to the basement, where a blue punching bag hung from one of the beams.

Boxing, my dad reckoned, was the best sport to teach a young boy. Not only would it keep him fit and in shape, it would teach him self-defense. Learning the art of boxing wasn't so that I could hurt others, however. And it wasn't really about making me a tough guy. Just as he wasn't an exceptional athlete, my dad wasn't really a tough guy—at least compared to the some of the other dads in the neighborhood who'd go out drinking on Saturday nights and get in fistfights with guys they'd known since grade school, only to make up a few hours later. It was very important in the neighborhood (and by extension, in life) to not take shit from anybody. Neighborhood logic went something like: "If you take shit, you aren't respected. And if you don't have respect, you don't have anything." So you'd better learn how to throw hands.

When I was about five, my dad and I went down to the basement for the first time to face that punching bag. There he would teach me (or at least try to teach me) about the mechanics of pugilism. The goal was that after two years of weekly sessions, I would be a lean, mean fighting machine.

My lessons lasted five weeks.

"The first step is learning how to throw a punch," my father said in the first week. "Let's see what you got." That was my cue to unleash a hail of mania and fury the likes of which that punching bag had never seen. I started punching with abandon, tiny fists flailing in rage, but after a while I got tired of the punching, and would kick, elbow, shoulder, and bite the big blue bag, while my dad stood nearby, smoking a cigarette and shaking his head. He had his work cut out for him.

Over the next few weeks, my dad tried to impart his boxing wisdom to me. *How you move your feet is just as important as how you use your hands. Be sure to properly follow through with your punches—you maximize your energy this way. Never buy cocaine from a man with one testicle. Make sure to twist your fist just slightly as your hand makes contact with his face—this tears the skin on impact. Learn to read your opponent's face and body language for the first sign of pain or weakness and take advantage of that. The man who invents a toilet for a motorcycle will become very rich, but will die alone. Boxing is 75 percent mental and 25 percent physical; street fighting is 90 percent intimidation and 10 percent ability. Determination trumps all.*

But there was just one problem: I didn't care about boxing. I didn't see any practical use for it. Whenever I got in fights with my friends, short skirmishes over toys or other stupid stuff, I followed a simple plan: Grab and squeeze until the other guy says "stop" or lay on top of him until he gives up. If I were on the losing end, this tactic would change to "Try not to let him hit you in the face. After he walks away, throw something at him and run into the house." Why then did I have to learn all this stuff about keeping my feet moving and using a frequent lazy jab to lull an opponent to sleep so that I could throw a thunderous combo? At the age of five, the only "combo" I cared to know about was a tube-shaped cracker filled with cheddar cheese.

So my interest in boxing quickly faded, if it ever existed at all. This was a crushing blow (no pun intended) to my father. He tried to show me the ropes of other sports, but I didn't take to them. I liked football, but it seemed too complicated, what with all the plays and different positions. I also liked to shoot hoops, but actual basketball games required way too much running. To this day, I still don't know how to skate, so no hockey. And no one played golf or soccer or any of those rich-people sports in my neighborhood; I don't even think I knew those sports existed until I went to high school.*

By the time I was six, and most likely because he figured I was a lost cause, my dad had given up teaching me about sports. Perhaps he realized that in order for me to truly become interested, it would have to happen organically. Or perhaps he was just lazy. Whichever, really.

But fortunately for him, there was one sport that I was drawn to on my own. What started as a passing interest grew first into an obsession and then into a lifelong love affair. After taking in a few games in person and on television, I made a simple decision: baseball was the greatest of all sports. And I wanted in.

Prior to actually playing Little League baseball, I was certain that Little League was simply the necessary first stop on my inevitable trip to the Baseball Hall of Fame. At the age of seven, I already had the rest of my life figured out, and Cooperstown was one of its last stops. After a successful stint in Little League, I'd move on to high school baseball, where I would break no less than six school records and be the first player in school history to start varsity all four years. My incredible baseball prow-

---

* Sort of like how when I first saw a horse, I thought it was just a really big dog. True story. Even though I admit I was pretty drunk on my twenty-second birthday.

ess would be responsible for my first sexual encounter, which would come during my freshman year after class in the biology lab with two sexually adventurous seniors: April, a redhead who bore a striking resemblance to Tawny Kitaen, and May, a blonde who bore a striking resemblance to any chick from any Poison video (or, I suppose, to one of the guys actually in Poison). They would pull me into the lab and ask, their breath sweet with green Life Savers, "So . . . what's your favorite month?" I'd look back at them slyly and say, "June." They'd laugh, but their laughter would dissolve into a hushed awe as they looked down at my bird, standing straight and proud in my baseball pants, which they would then take and do whatever it was that girls did with guys' birds (I hadn't figured that part out yet). Then they would tell the rest of the school what an incredible lover I was, and the remainder of my time in high school would be filled with make-out sessions and masterfully unhooked bras, perfect grades and perfect SATs, and game-winning hits and adoration, adoration, adoration.

Of course, my mother would cry at graduation when, during my valedictorian speech, I announced that I was turning down the big baseball schools and instead choosing the academic scholarship to Harvard, where I could both make her proud in the classroom and lead their once-proud but now-faltering baseball program back to glory. And of course, that is exactly what I would do. After an 0-28 season the year before, the team would finish with a 26-2 record in my freshman year (one loss coming when I had to play the entire outfield by myself because my teammates were involved in a minor bus accident and the other when I was momentarily hampered with dysentery; even in my fantasies I was a hypochondriac). We would never lose again on my watch.

After my freshman year, the Phillies, Yankees, Mets, Red Sox, and pretty much every major-league team would come calling with offers of big money, fast cars, and loose women. But I'd brush them all aside because I had another dream to attend to first. In addition to being a stellar athlete, I'd be an equally stellar student. And for my honors thesis, I'd have an ambitious goal to perform the first ever heart-liver double transplant—*in front of a live studio audience*. It would be a success, and afterward three girls would make out with me at the same time, thus concluding my college career.

And then on to the majors. You know how the rest of the story goes. First overall pick by the hometown Philadelphia Phillies. A rookie year featuring the Rookie of the Year Award and a World Series championship, earning me the nickname Jason "Midas" Mulgrew, since everything I touched turned to gold. Then sixteen Gold Gloves, eight MVP awards (the writers would eventually turn against me), almost 800 home runs, and a career .340 average. Later, I'd be up there on the podium at the Hall of Fame, giving my speech. It would be similar to the speech that I'd given to the Nobel Prize people only a year before, but more about baseball and less about peace/medicine/literature/physics/general awesomeness. I'd look at my mom and dad and thank them for all their support over the years. They'd smile and nod with appreciation, and then look at my brother (the convict) and my sister (the telemarketer) and shake their heads in disapproval. Then I'd look at my wife, Cindy Crawford, and thank her for always being there for me, through all the wins and losses, slumps and hitting streaks. She'd smile and wink, and I'd blush. Then Cindy and I would go back to the hotel and do whatever it was that a guy and a girl did when they were in a hotel room together.

So surely I would take to Little League very quickly. This wasn't even in question. I had never played fast-pitch hardball before, but I wasn't concerned with this.

No one I knew played fast-pitch hardball, because that required resources that we didn't have access to. For one thing, grass and open space were both pretty hard to come by on Second Street. If we were feeling ambitious, my friends and I could head down to "the Rec,"* the park down at Third and Shunk that had two baseball fields, some basketball courts, a public pool, and a lot of grass. But going to the Rec was a ballsy move, because we ran the risk of being hassled or picked on by older kids or some of the Puerto Rican or black kids from the surrounding neighborhoods. I loved baseball, but I loved not getting wedgies and not having to run from a large group of Puerto Rican kids who wanted my glove even more.

Instead, as city kids, we improvised, playing various baseball-type games that were easier and more accessible to us. There were five variations:

- Wiffle ball: This was played in a schoolyard with as little as two players with your standard Wiffle ball

---

* It wasn't until I was about seventeen that I realized that the proper spelling was "the Rec," short for "the Recreation Center." Previously, I had always assumed that it was "the Wreck," because of the sketchiness of the people who hung out there and the disrepair of the fields, courts, and pool.

and yellow bat. There were no bases. One strike and you were out, three outs per inning. Anything over the fence was a home run; anything that got past the pitcher was a single; anything successfully fielded (even a grounder) was an out. Play until you have to go home or your arms fall off. Keep score dutifully. Most likely fight with opponent about the score.

- Stickball: Similar to Wiffle ball with three differences: 1) played with stick and rubber ball; 2) a strike zone is drawn behind the hitter against the wall of the school, and the hitter now has three strikes per out; 3) fighting over scoring more intense than in Wiffle ball, due to the more fast-paced nature of the game.

- Halfball: Same as stickball, but played with a tennis ball cut in half. My least favorite baseball-derived game. (Why would anyone cut a perfectly good tennis ball in half?)

- Streetball: Played with full teams in the street/school-yard, with bases drawn in chalk on the asphalt/cement. Like real baseball, except with tennis ball and loaded Wiffle-ball bat (a Wiffle-ball bat cut open, stuffed with newspapers, and taped up). Also unlike real baseball in that someone's mildly retarded younger brother will be required to play and a fight will usually break out between the older nonretarded brother and the younger somewhat-retarded brother. Hilarity will ensue, Sunny Delight will be consumed, purple stuff will be eschewed.

- Killball: Like streetball, but a mix of 90 percent base-

ball and 10 percent dodgeball. A hitter can be called
out if the fielder catches his ball, throws it at him, and
hits him with it when he is not on base. It was with the
birth of this game that many of us realized that our testicles were sensitive things to be respected, rather than
decorations dangling below our penises.

I spent the early part of my youth playing these games re-
ligiously. By the time an opportunity to play in Little League
presented itself, I felt like I was ready to take that next step.

Yet I don't want to give the impression that I was just some
kid playing the game because he had nothing else to do or because playing Little League is just what you're supposed to do
as a kid. I loved baseball—a lot—not just to play, but to watch
and enjoy as well. Every day I'd pore over the sports section of
the *Daily News*, analyzing the box scores, noting how many hits
Mike Schmidt had, whether or not Juan Samuel had stolen a
base, or if Steve Bedrosian had picked up the save. I collected
baseball cards with a frightening obsession/compulsion that
would meet its equal later in my life only when a) I discovered
masturbating; b) I discovered getting drunk; and c) I discovered sex.* Collecting baseball cards was not just a hobby, it was a
lifestyle. My mom inadvertently ruined the second half of 1988
for me when she got me some lame-ass OshKosh B'gosh over-
alls for my birthday instead of the Donruss-brand Jose Canseco
rookie card that I so desperately wanted.** I spent hours lust-

---

* In that order—and sadly, great stretches of time passed between the three.
** In retrospect, a great call on my mom's part. Back then, this card cost about

ing after prized cards in Lou's Cards & Comics on Broad Street and whole afternoons and evenings in my room studying the statistics on the backs of the cards. If you had asked me how many hits Wade Boggs had in 1983, how many home runs Dale Murphy hit in 1985, or how many strikeouts Doc Gooden had in his rookie year, I could tell you instantly.* If I had put half as much effort into schoolwork as I did studying these cards, I would have graduated from grade school in four years and would now probably be a Ph.D. touring the country lecturing on the reproductive habits of the cnidarians of the South Pacific. Instead it took me eight whole years to graduate and now I couldn't tell you which president is on the twenty-dollar bill.** Stupid baseball obsession.

I wasn't just a stat nerd; I watched a lot of games, too. Baseball became my first love in large part because it was (and still is) the most accessible of sports. First and foremost, there are 162 freaking games, double that of hockey and basketball and ten times that of football, allowing for plenty of time to get familiar with the sport. Not only that, the bulk of baseball is played during the summer, when kids all over the country are off from school and driving their parents crazy by telling them things like "Dad, it's a long story, but the air conditioner caught on fire" and "Mom, I'm not sure how it happened, but Dennis

---

forty dollars. Using our special currency converter, we know that forty dollars to a nine year-old is roughly equivalent to $680 to an adult. As of this writing, this card is going for about two dollars on eBay.

* 210, 37, and 276 (!), respectively. And yes, I had to look that up. But back then I wouldn't have had to. Trust me.
** Andrew Jackson. I had to look that up, too.

is gone—can you make me another little brother?" as soon as they get home from work. So when not being tremendous pains in the asses, my friends and I enjoyed nothing more than sitting in front of the television watching the Philadelphia Phillies play some of the worst baseball in the major leagues. And we had ample time to do so.

My friends and I were also lucky because we lived just over a mile away from Veterans Stadium, the home of the Phillies. A general admission ticket to a Phillies game was only four bucks and you couldn't get much more adventurous than you and your friends trekking all the way up the Vet to take in a game—without adults. My buddies and I would head to an afternoon game, buy our cheap tickets, and then spend the first third of the game trying to move closer to the field and sneak into better seats. Fortunately, this was easy to do, as, like I said, the Phils weren't exactly packing them in at the time with their high-quality play. Then we'd sit and watch, taking it all in, basking in the glow of America's great pastime. This was the ultimate for us, sitting in the stands, the sun, the heat making our hair matted with sweat under our cheap mesh Phillies hats. It was such a grown-up thing to do—"We're going to the Vet to catch a ball game"—but also so easy. And because baseball imbued us with such a great sense of responsibility at such a young age, we repaid the sport with our fierce loyalty.

Loyalty or not, the Phillies stunk. The roster of players that passed through the teams during this time was laughable, but there was one Phillie who stood above all others. A man whose push-broom mustache teemed with virility and strength. A man whose presence in a powder-blue Phillies uniform would inspire a generation of young kids to try to knock one out of the park. His name was Michael Jack Schmidt. And he was my idol.

Mike Schmidt's career was winding down by the time I began to get into baseball (though I did get to appreciate some of his good years toward the end there, like his MVP season in 1986). But Schmidt was the first athlete that I was aware of who transcended his sport. He was not only the best player in baseball in the 1980s, he had so woven himself into the fabric of Philadelphia, a city to which he had helped bring a championship, that each time he came to the plate it was not an at-bat but actually an *experience* that garnered a combination of respect, awe, and gratitude from the fans. And then, if he struck out, the fans would boo the shit out of him. Hell, even if he didn't strike out, we'd *still* boo the shit out of him. We might have loved him, but hey, we were still Philly fans. Remember—we're the ones who threw snowballs at Santa Claus (because he was drunk), batteries at J. D. Drew (because he was a prick who refused to sign with the team when drafted by them), and applauded Michael Irvin of the Dallas Cowboys when he lay on the turf of the Vet with a potentially serious spinal injury (because, well, he's Michael Irvin).

Because of old number 20, the final piece of the puzzle for Little League was set: I would play third base, just like Schmidty. I would also grow a mustache like him, but that might take some time. For now, I had the experience, the love, the knowledge, and the plan. But every superstar has to start somewhere, so in the spring of 1987 I hopped into my dad's truck and we went the orientation meeting for Sabres Youth League Baseball. My destiny awaited. My time had come. Play ball.

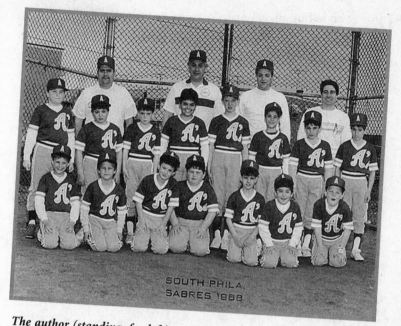

The author (standing, far left) and his teammates prepare for another grueling season of McDonald's and talking about masturbating.

It started fortuitously enough. After signing up, I was assigned to a team, the A's, and given a uniform just like the green and yellow one that the Oakland A's had, so I looked the part of a big-league player. Not only that, I was able to procure the number 20, the same number worn by Mike Schmidt himself. I overlooked the fact that it was the only number left in my size and attributed this coincidence to fate. The gods were smiling upon me. This was going to be great.

[*dramatic pause with DUM-DUM-DUMMM music*]

Well, at least that's what I thought.

I ended up playing two seasons in Little League. If I had a baseball card, my stats could be broken down as follows:

- Games played: 25 (out of a possible 26)
- Team record with me: 0-25
- Team record without me: 1-0
- Number of at-bats: 75
- Hits: 1
- Number of times my bat made contact with a pitch: 3
- Number of times the contact my bat made with a pitch was accidental: 3
- Doubles: 0
- Triples: 0
- Home runs: 0
- Walks: 8
- Number of times hit by pitch: 6
- Number of times I cried after being hit by a pitch: 11
- Number of times I cried for other reasons (no more barbecue potato chips, my batting helmet is too small, I'm missing the Balki show, etc.): 22
- Pepsis consumed: 148
- Number of times masturbation discussed on the bench: 512
- Number of times those discussing masturbation had actually masturbated: 0.5 (Once our second baseman admitted that he rubbed his sister's friend's bra on his bird, so we gave him half credit. The rest of us said that we had masturbated, but of course we were lying.)

To be clear, my failings in Little League were no fault of my own. I had both the drive and the talent (I swear), but I was cut down before I could bring any of this to the surface. Like many Little Leaguers, my biggest fear was the ball, that little white sphere that was capable of such tremendous damage as a bruise or red mark. This fear doomed me almost immediately. In one of our first practices, we had drills to determine who would play where. In a very un-despot-like fashion, Coach Mike asked each of us where we wanted to play. I was dismayed when I and about six other kids picked third base, but I let it slide because I was obviously far superior to these mongrels. The A's third baseman would be determined by audition. You had to stand at third, field a grounder hit to you by one of the assistant coaches, and throw it over to first.

I was entirely unprepared for this. There was no warm-up, no explanation, no nothing. This was the first time I'd ever faced live hardball hitting, and it was enough to make me crap my pants (which I'm pretty sure I did at a game at some point during my career). But there was no time to worry here, since Coach Mike, seeing my number 20, called me up to be first in the audition. I crouched in a defensive position, trying to keep my poise. A very short time later—think a second divided by about two million—the grounder sprung off the assistant coach's bat toward me.

I have heard athletes in interviews talk about how when they're playing at the top of their game, everything moves very slowly—they achieve a heightened sense of awareness and can see holes in the defensive line or the basket looks as big as an ocean or the fastball looks like it's coming to the plate in slow motion.

But there was nothing slow about this moment. The grounder came at me like a torpedo—an angry white meteor seemingly shot from a rocket launcher—and took a hard bounce in front of me, before popping me square on the right shin. It happened so quickly that I couldn't even brace myself for the ball's impact. Being a pussy, I went down into a crumpled heap, made a sound similar to a piglet falling down a flight of stairs, and hemmed and hawed about how my leg was broken. The coaches helped me off the field to the bench where I could rest up and eat cookies. Welcome to Little League, dickhead.

I'll can the suspense and tell you that I didn't pass the audition. Instead of starring at third base, I spent my first season in right field, and when in my second season the designated hitter was instituted, I was my team's DH. This suited me just fine, as it allowed me more time to sit on the bench and talk about masturbation, but it also meant I was 99 percent sure that I wasn't going to win any Gold Glove awards. Oh, well.

As for my team life, I couldn't field, run, hit, or even dress myself properly, but it didn't matter. Put me in a uniform, give me an audience and all the Mountain Dew I can drink, and I'll survive and thrive. The good news for me was that the whole team sucked, so we didn't care much about the glory of the sport. Through all the losses and consolation trips to McDonald's, I learned that my teammates were a strange group of kids who proved themselves to be endless sources of entertainment. Little League teams are a lot like the Seven Dwarfs, as each kid on the team has a certain unique personality. The sum of these personalities constitutes your average Little League team:

- The Coach's Son (3B): Why else would a man coach a Little League team unless his son is playing on that team? The Coach's Son can take any number of personalities mentioned below, but on my team he was just a little slow. Or perhaps I'm just jealous, because of course he wanted—and was awarded—my position, third base. I don't think I'm bitter anymore though. I'm a writer now, so I get, like, a ton of blow jobs.

- The Eight-Year-Old Who's Really Nineteen (1B): Mancuso. That was his name on my team. You know the type: he's the best player on the team and has had pubes since before you were born; while the other players are talking about candy he's complaining about his mortgage; and he has to miss a few games here and there for jury duty. My memory is a little blurry, but I'm fairly certain Mancuso would show up to games on a motorcycle, hit a home run every time he came up to the plate, and then speed away, surely to go smoke cigarettes and have sex with his girlfriend or possibly wife. Meanwhile, I'd go home, eat a pouch of powdered cheese, and throw up. How was it possible that this guy and I were on the same team?

- The Eight-Year-Old Who's Really Four (OF): On the opposite end of the spectrum, I'm sure I saw this kid eating baby food on at least one occasion. He required a special bat that was lighter than the others, as well as a smaller helmet, probably taken from the tee-ball kids. To his credit, he was an on-base machine. Since it was impossible to throw him a strike (since due to his size his strike zone was the size of an apple) and he was too weak and underdeveloped to actually swing the bat, he was guaranteed to walk. And in Little League, we learn that a walk is just as good as a single.

- The Fat Kid (C): In my first year, we had the real deal— a solid 150-pounder named Larry, who looked like ten pounds of shit in a five-pound bag in his skintight uniform. He rarely played, preferring instead to sit on the bench to eat sandwiches and drink chocolate milk. He was a magnificent son of a bitch and my best friend on the team and I was crushed when he didn't return in my second year. We assumed he either had a heart attack or ate himself, but these rumors could neither be confirmed nor disconfirmed.

- The Gay Kid (SS): On my team, we called him "Hollywood." He was our shortstop and had a flair for the dramatic. I would not be surprised if today he were involved in some capacity in an off-off-Broadway production of Chekhov's The Seagull, performed entirely by mimes in drag.

- The Kid Who Is Definitely Abused at Home (OF): Usually, this kid sits at the end of the bench, looking sad and being silent. More often than not he is ridiculed, but the kid who fit this description on my team was not, since we knew he was a little too screwy to be messed with. And that's all I have to say about this, since this kid has probably grown into a very deviant adult more than capable of stabbing me in the parking lot of my local Home Depot.

• The Total Prick (2B): Usually the second-best player on the team, aside from the kid who's really nineteen. However, unlike the kid who's really nineteen, who is too cool (or tired from being up all night with his fussy newborn) to come down on or yell at his teammates for their poor play, this guy is very vocal about his teammates' suckiness. This kid is despised by the rest of team and more than likely has a hot mom. He also usually has a dickhead name like Chad, Brock, or Lance.

• The Kid Whose Dad Will Punch Him in the Face if He Fucks Up (P): Since we sucked, my team was bereft of such a player, but I saw my fair share of these guys in Little League. I recall one game in which the opposing pitcher gave up a bases-clearing double, and then his father, an assistant coach, plied himself from the bench to go out to the mound and smack and yell at his son for a solid four minutes as players and parents stood in horror. His father walked off the mound and the kid continued pitching through tears. When he hit the next kid with a fastball that came in at about 106 miles per hour and then struck out the following kid who was too concerned with not getting hit to swing the bat, his dad greeted him as he came off the field, shouting, "See? That's what I'm talking about! Good job!" I remember seeing this and feeling grateful that my dad didn't come to games. I'd take a "no show" dad over a "beat you in front of your friends after a double and leave you crying on the mound" dad any day of the week, thank you very much.

If I had a personality, I'd be "the Entertainer," the guy who sucks but who doesn't care and has a good time with it. He may have low self-esteem, have a strange home life, or be confused about his sexuality (not that, um, *I* was like this), so he can take on shades of each personality. He will usually grow up and either be named Mid-Atlantic Salesman of the Year or die of a cocaine-induced heart attack at age thirty-one. So I guess I should start selling something, and quickly.

It was in Little League during my tenure as Team Jester that I learned an important life lesson. Self-deprecation can make you many a friend. I was the worst guy on the team, but like everything else in my life, I learned to spin this to my advantage, offering myself as the butt of endless jokes in exchange for being well liked. I saw that you can make those around you feel better about themselves by making light of the fact that you're not as good/athletic/handsome/skinny/straight as they are. It was at this time that the Joke was perfected. In Little League, the Joke sounded like: "Nice grab out there in center, Billy. If that rocket had been hit to me, I'd have to ask you guys to start collecting napkins so I could clean off the shit trickling down my leg!" In high school, when a friend had to help me with car trouble, the Joke had evolved into something like: "Damn, Steve—you're like a real man with this car repair stuff. Here you are fixing a carburetor and I don't even know how to pump gas. I usually just open the hood and spray the shit everywhere." In college while drunk at parties, I would use the Joke to routinely refer to my tiny penis in front of women—comparing it to a thumb, wine cork, button, light switch, acorn, and pen cap, among other things—in the hopes that if any of these women actually saw my penis and saw that it wasn't quite that small, they'd be pleasantly surprised.*

Playing youth baseball didn't teach me about teamwork, honor, discipline, respect, or responsibility. Nor, as evinced by my .013 average, had I learned any physical skill, since I was fucking terrible and there was no way around that. It didn't teach me confidence, either, since there is not much dignity in repeatedly failing in front of your peers. Instead I learned about resilience: how to deal with problems and how to cope in less than ideal situations. I couldn't make contact with the ball if it was on a tee, but at least I had all the Rice Krispies treats I could eat. I learned about humility; how unfounded confidence can be a detriment. I wasn't going to break any home run records, but maybe I could make it through the rest of the season without crying (although I usually failed in this). And I learned humor; *everything* is funny. Yeah, I suck at baseball and I just struck out, but I think I gave myself a fucking hernia in the process. And it could always be worse—at least I'm not that kid on the Warriors who had a wet dream in the outfield.

---

* Although most women who saw my penis in college were usually too drunk to take notice anyway. That, or they were fast asleep and so unable to see it pressed against the glass of their dorm room window.

I still continued to watch and enjoy baseball after my spectacular failure in Little League. I don't think my love for baseball could be altered by anything, say, even if I learned that all those stats that I so revered as a kid—Mike Schmidt's 548 career home runs, Roger Maris's single-season record of 61 homers, Hank Aaron's 755 career home runs—were being threatened or surpassed by a generation of juiced-up meatheads with tiny balls. Sometimes you just have to stay loyal.

And today, though I don't even play in beer leagues because just hearing my coworkers talk about them makes me tired, I still spend whole mornings and afternoons studying statistics, but no longer are they on the back of cards. The name of my game is fantasy baseball, which occupies about 75 percent of my time at work from March until October every year. I am happy to say that all the success I was unable to achieve in Little League or in the majors I have found in fantasy baseball, where, as commissioner of the prestigious Iron Sheik league, I have won four of the past eight championships. Mike Schmidt, I could never be. But if Mike had a nerdy brother who was really into numbers and really afraid of girls, well, I could probably be him.

Chapter Six

On the Relationship Between Genetics and Hustling

My Grandpop Brennan won every cruise ship dance contest he entered. He had the trophies to prove it, too. They lined the walls of the basement, mementos of his excellence on the dance floor. He was very proud of them and his dancing abilities. He had no training, either, something he never neglected to mention. Despite being a chubby Irish guy, he could just *move*.* It was innate. The only downside to his victories was that he could not share in their glory with his wife, Isabel. Not because she passed away or because they were divorced or anything tragic like that, but because she wasn't as good a dancer as he was. She

---

* I believe in some circles this would be known as "blue-eyed soul."

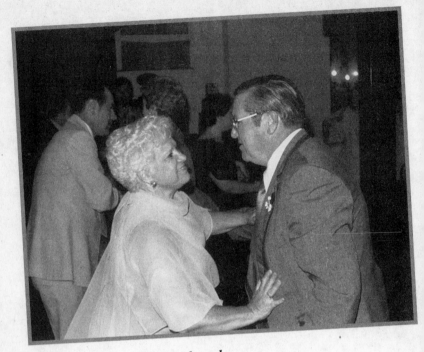

The danciest dancers that ever danced.

was no slouch, but dancing was not her forte in the same way that it was my grandfather's. She knew this, accepted it, and was "fine" with it. On the cruise ships my grandfather would enter these competitions with the girls who worked in the clubs on the ship. The two of them would cut their proverbial rug and ace the competition, and after each victory my grandfather would present the trophy to my grandmother, dedicating it to her. Then she'd tell him jokingly, but maybe only half jokingly, to stick the trophy up his ass.

I never got to know my grandfather. He died in 1984 at the age of fifty-six, a few months before my fifth birthday. I have few memories of him. One was that he always brought me Kit-Kats. I loved, and still love, Kit-Kats. That special combination of wafers, nougat, and chocolate cast a spell on me at an early age, and I have my grandfather to thank for that. By extension, I could also blame him for my lifelong weight problem, but I think I'll leave that alone for now.

The other memory of my grandfather I have is going drinking with him. This was just after my brother was born in 1983. My grandfather would come around the house, pick me up, and take me out to give my mom some peace. Then grandpop and I

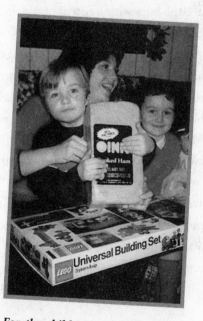

For the child who has everything: Legos and a block of "Oink" ham (stipend for later-in-life therapy not included).

would hit the bars. I'd get a Coke and he'd get a grown-up drink (always a Manhattan) and I'd watch him go around and talk to everyone in the bar, hamming it up one moment, having whispered discussions to the side the next, pats on the backs and handshakes all around. Meanwhile, I sat there occupying myself with the plastic sword-shaped drink stirrers, which I would use as weapons for my GI Joe guys, which I would bring along on these trips to keep myself occupied. After a bit, we'd head to another bar and the scene would repeat itself. By the time we were finished, I'd have pockets full of these little swords and a belly full of Coke.[*]

I'd also leave the bars with a fistful of money. All the older guys my grandpop talked to would make a fuss over me, messing my hair, calling me "champ," saying things like, "Jasper, how are you doing in school?" or "Hey, Jasper, how about them Phillies?" These men always called me Jasper, likely because my own grandfather also called me Jasper. For some reason, Grandpop Brennan had a bit of trouble with the name Jason, which in the early '80s was relatively new (or newly popular). So when my grandpop would introduce me to a friend as "my grandson Jasper," I'd have to correct him and say, "No, Grandpop—it's *Jason*, not Jasper!" Grandpop would take a sip of his Manhattan, laugh it off, slap me on the back, and say, "That's what I said! You'd better take that fudge out of your ears!"[**] Possibly because they felt bad that my grandpop continually screwed up

---

* The kid kind, not the now kind.
** Or he could get the name right. I didn't have no dang fudge in my ears.

my name, the older guys I'd get introduced to as Jasper/Jason always ended each hello by giving me a dollar bill and buying me a soda. Since we'd go to several bars an afternoon, I'd end up with ten or so dollars. Not a bad haul for a four-year-old, so I was able to find it in my heart to forgive both them and my grandpop for calling me Jasper. Then I'd return home to my mom and wreak havoc, since I had just had thirteen Cokes in four hours.

I loved these trips to the bars, both going on them as a child and reliving them in my memory when I got older. Until a few years ago, I thought these drinking sessions with my grandfather were his way of bonding with me. Sure, maybe it's not entirely healthy to bring a child to a bar, let him watch you drink, then drunkenly drive him around to several other bars, then drop him off at his parents' house so hopped up on caffeine that he'd run screaming through the house with his pants off yelling that he was the Lizard King. But in a strange, semidysfunctional way, there was something sweet about the whole thing; a grandfather getting his grandson prepared for the lifestyle that he would take to so readily later in his own life. Kind of nice, isn't it?

But then I got older and I realized that the original intention of these trips was not to bond. Nor was it to prepare me for later life. My grandfather was out "collecting." And he was using me as a decoy.

After serving as a chef in the merchant marine in World War II, my Grandpop Brennan, like all the other men in the neighborhood, became a longshoreman.* When he wasn't cooking, a longshoreman was basically what he was in the merchant marine, assisting the navy by transporting goods and supplies, so the transition to civilian life was easier for him than many. But working longshore was just his day job, a legitimate way to pay the bills. He had other, more interesting pursuits.

My grandfather was a number writer. This was the job for which he was known all throughout the neighborhood. Number writing is an old-school form of gambling. Though it still exists, it's a dying art, slowly being fazed out by the rampant sports gambling of today. Back in the old days, the state lottery system didn't exist. So organized crime took it upon itself to create one. Number writing is an intensely complicated (and secretive) type of gambling. Whole books can be written about it.** But I'll give it to you in a couple of paragraphs.

The one-sentence explanation is that number writing is essentially a private lottery run by organized crime. I am hesitant to use the term *organized crime,* as it conjures up images of burly Italian guys in bad suits. But it's the term to use because a) number writing was (and is) highly organized, and b) it is illegal. You would play numbers like you play the lottery today, but instead of going to a machine, you'd go to a guy like my grandpop. He'd take down your number and how much you

---

* I often wondered why he didn't open a restaurant after serving as a chef in the war, but then I realized that he probably wasn't making paupiette of black sea bass in a barolo sauce in the service, and South Philly was already full of places that serve shit on a shingle and other mysterious (but delicious) foodstuffs.

** Whole books probably *have* been written about it, but that would require research, which, as mentioned, is not my thing.

wanted to bet. For example, 789 every day for two dollars. The winning number is not determined by drawing with numbered Ping-Pong balls but by horse races. The first digit of the three-digit winning number would be based on the winners of a certain number of the races. For example, let's say that in the first three races of the day at X Racetrack, Horse 2 wins the first race, Horse 6 wins the second, and Horse 1 wins the third. These three numbers (2-6-1) would be taken and put into a mysterious mathematical formula resulting in a single, one-digit number. That single, one-digit number would be the first digit of the day's three-digit winning number. The process would be repeated, where Races 4–5–6 would provide the second winning digit and Races 7–8–9 the third.

The "bank" or "backer" is the man who announces the day's winning number. This is a man who is fairly high up in the system and, as the name implies, fronts the money (he could either be the end of the line or someone could front money to him, leading further and further up a hierarchy). He then would call his bookies, sitting in bars all over the neighborhood, who would then relay the winning number to his "clients," the people "in his book."* My grandfather started as a bookie-level number writer, then became a backer. It was a profession that suited him, as it required him to do his two favorite things: be social and drink. Since he was very, very

---

* The formula was not so secret that people didn't know it. If you sit at a bar today, you might notice an old-timer screaming "Oh shit!" in disgust after a race. It could be because of his horse, but it could be because he just realized that his number wasn't coming out that day, since he had computed at least one digit of the winning number after the race.

good at these two things, he became very, very good at being a number writer.

This side business allowed my grandfather to provide a good life for his wife and six kids. My father, who grew up on powdered milk and didn't have a steak until he was on his honeymoon, always called my mom "rich" for her seemingly opulent childhood, which included annual family vacations down the shore and more than one toy on Christmas. And while the money was good, the excitement of knowing that Daddy was a popular bookie made it even better. My mom speaks almost fondly of a time when she was eight years old and their house was raided by a squadron of undercover vice cops. My grandfather and his partner were upstairs when it started—the photos on the walls shaking as the police kicked down the door. Inside, six children ranging in age from one to fifteen sat dumbfounded when the police burst into the home. As the police rushed upstairs to apprehend my grandpop, he came out of the bedroom and surrendered. But before being taken away, he asked if he could get his kids out of the house—he didn't want them to see their father being led away in handcuffs. The police agreed, so my grandfather went and said good-bye to his kids—Mikey, Joey, Kathy, Anne, Maureen, and the baby, Billy. He gave each a kiss and promised them everything would be all right, but to Billy he gave something else—his scripts of numbers. The numbers were always written on rice paper so that they could dissolve quickly if they needed to be flushed down the toilet. My grandfather had stuffed them down his pants when he heard the raid coming, and now he removed them and stuck them in Billy's diaper. If they had been confiscated in the raid, not only would it have been proof of his involvement in gambling, but he also would have had to pay out hundreds or even thousands of dollars in lost bets. The kids were taken from the house, moved only a block away by my grandmother to my grandfather's sister's house, my Great-Aunt Mary. When Mary discovered the numbers stuffed in Billy's diaper, she panicked and—sure enough—flushed them down the toilet. My grandfather was released after a night in jail, and his first order of business was to go around to Mary's house to pick up the numbers. When she told him that she had panicked and flushed them, he got so enraged that he didn't speak to his sister for over a year, so upset was he that he had to pay out all that money.

So when my grandpop took me out on these bar trips, he was, more or less, using me. That's not to say that he didn't like showing me off to his friends and acquaintances, nor is it to say that we didn't have a good time (see: GI Joes, Cokes, plastic drink stirrers), but my primary purpose was to serve as a decoy. I was there to throw off suspicion from the cops who regularly harassed him. If he were alone, he'd look more like he was making the rounds. If he had his grandson with him, he was just showing the kid off. * He did the same to my mother and her brothers and sisters when they were kids, so when I was old enough, I became one of the next generation of decoys.

More than a number writer, my grandfather was a true street entrepreneur who always had a scheme or a plan and was never

---

* I'm still not sure why this makes sense. I would think that a grown man taking a child in and out of bars all day would arouse more suspicion than if he went sans child, but when I pressed my family about this, their only response was "It was different back then."

afraid to have someone in the family involved. When his son, my Uncle Joey, got a job as a teenager at the local supermarket, my grandpop would head down during Joey's shift and "buy" turkeys, hams, and meat, then take them and sell them down at the waterfront to his coworkers and longshoremen buddies. The same happened when my mom worked at Toys 'R' Us when I was a kid. As a kid, having a mom that works for Toys 'R' Us is the equivalent of me now marrying a brewer or someone who owns an onion ring factory. I had a direct connection to Shangri-la, and I was crushed when she finally quit to take another job. It was worse than learning there was no Santa. If he had lived to see it, my grandfather would have been crushed when she quit, too, since he was using her in the same way that he was using my Uncle Joey. Especially around Christmastime, my grandpop would go to Toys 'R' Us during my mom's shift, fill up his cart, and wait patiently to be checked out by her, even if other lines were shorter. She'd scan every second or third item, my grandfather would pay, and then take the toys straight down the waterfront for resale. In this way, he was like a modern-day Robin Hood. Well, not really, but it sounds kinda nice.

That was my grandfather, street entrepreneur, number writer, fun son of a bitch. Wheeling, dealing, always having a good time, and perhaps influencing me more than either he or I knew.

Like many young boys, I was fascinated with fireworks. What's not to like, really? Let's see, there are explosions (check), noise (check), light (check), and the potential for extreme finger-losing danger (check, check, check). One of my favorite times of the year was when the Phillies would have their annual early July home stand to coincide with the July Fourth holiday. Each night, over three games, the sky above Veterans Stadium would be filled with exploding light: the flares of the reds and blues and greens dancing above our heads.

My mom and dad (or one or the other) always took me and my brother and sister to see these fireworks. We'd drive up to the Lakes, the park that neighbored the Vet, and make a nice little evening of it. My friends would be there with their parents, and so we'd run around, play Wiffle ball, and carry on. Meanwhile, our parents would talk, drink beer, and barbecue while listening to the game on the radio. One of the dads would announce that the game was over, and my friends and I would fix our attention on the night sky, hoping to be the first to see the opening flare of the light darting upward from the stadium.

And then, with a sonic boom, it began; our heads pointed skyward to catch the show of noise and light. I'd sit there silent, neck arched, mesmerized by the display. The sulfur burning off from the fireworks, mixed with the smell of the grass and the grilled meat; the blasts of light reflecting off the car windshields, parked on the grass with their hatchbacks and truck beds open; the humidity and the thin layer of mist that hung on me like a cloak; the booms and *ooohs* drowning out the sound of Harry Kalas and Richie Ashburn on the Phillies postgame show coming from the radio—these are some of the finest memories of my youth.

As I grew older, I learned that fireworks didn't just come in the sky-exploding variety. I knew about firecrackers but didn't consider them fireworks, since all they did was make loud noises and blow shit up. I was totally behind the blowing-shit-up aspect of the firecrackers, but what most interested me were projectile fireworks, such as bottle rockets, which could be fired at people and stray animals; light fireworks, like jumping jacks, which looked like firecrackers but instead spun noiselessly in a ball of light; and my favorite, the Roman candle, which combined the best aspects of the bottle rocket and the jumping jack, as it could be fired at people and stray animals with much more accuracy than the bottle rocket and would light up brighter than any jumping jack.*

But these fireworks, though awesome, were hard to come by. We only got see them on the Fourth of July when our parents lit them (we were never allowed to even get near them, let alone fire them off). Otherwise, we were fireworks-less 364 days a year. Until I met Henry.

The idea for the fireworks business was mine. Let's be clear about that right away. David will tell you that he was the mastermind behind our enterprise, but that is simply not the truth. I won't belittle his contributions to the business, because they were indeed significant, but it was my brainchild. All mine.

Now we can move forward.

After my parents' divorce was finalized, my mom, brother,

---

* For the record, I have never and would never use any sort of firework on an animal, stray or domesticated. Not only because this would be cruel, but because if I missed, the animal would probably be pretty pissed off and come after me. No thanks.

sister, and I moved back into our old house and my dad moved out. He bounced around a few different places before settling down in what had been his brother Mikey's house. The house was on a street called Beulah Street, which at the time was not a nice part of the neighborhood. However, despite this, or perhaps more appropriately, *because of* this, the street was like a family. The good people of the block banded together to create a safer environment for their families, resulting in a true sense of community.

One of the members of this community was a guy named Henry, who lived across the street from my dad. A middle-aged Italian guy who smoked three packs a day, Henry delivered pizzas in the neighborhood for my favorite pizza place, Two Street Pizza. But Henry's real passion was not pizza. It was fireworks—glorious, glorious fireworks. Shortly after my dad and Henry made acquaintances, no doubt having bonded over their mutual love of and admiration for Marlboro Reds, my dad took me over to Henry's house and into his basement. I was around eleven at the time, young, impressionable, and always looking for new ways to hurt myself and/or get in trouble. And then I saw Henry's basement.

The basement was filled with fireworks. And I mean *filled* in the most literal sense—there was not two square feet of space that wasn't covered by some sort of fireworks. All I saw before me were mounds of mounds of packages, Chinese lettering, and crinkly red paper. Henry had all the normal fireworks that I enjoyed, but in quantities I had never seen before: cases of bricks of jumping jacks, firecrackers, Roman candles, and bottle rockets, stacked on top of each other, several rows deep. He walked carefully around the room, pointing out and explaining to me the fireworks that I was unfamiliar with. But I was too dazed to notice. I had found where I wanted to spend the rest of my life.

These were the years that my dad was still feeling guilty about the divorce, so I walked out of Henry's basement with more fireworks than I could carry—surely enough to last me for the next few months.

(I'd be back for more in a week.)

The next day, I took some of my fireworks around the Park, the concrete playground where my friends and I hung out at the corner of Second and Jackson. Once night fell, I pulled some of the jumping jacks out of my pocket and lit them with matches I had taken from my house. In that very instant, I transformed from "that nerdy kid who I hear kisses his hamster" to "Holy shit, that guy has fireworks!" Remember, we were just kids at this point, in only fourth or fifth grade. Fireworks are to fifth-graders what sex is to high school kids: mysterious, tantalizing, and terrifying. Also, highly addictive.

After the display was over, a display which consisted of me gingerly lighting single jumping jacks and throwing them as far away from me as possible so as not to get hurt, my friend Jimmy the Muppet came up to me.

"Yo, you got any more of them?" he asked.

"Yeah, I got some more at home, but I ain't bringing them out." The last thing I needed was for everyone to make a big deal over the fireworks. Don't get me wrong—I liked the idea of the uptick in popularity that being the proud owner and displayer of fireworks would no doubt produce, but if my friends knew how many I had, they'd be hitting me up for free packs. And the older kids ... forget about it. If they knew I was holding fireworks, I'd be beat up and picked on into oblivion and left without a single bottle rocket to my name. So I intended to ration them out, using only a pack here and there, and preferably when no older kids were around.

"I don't want you to bring them out—I want to buy some off you."

Jimmy and I snuck away from the crowd and I took him around to my house, where after promising him not to tell anyone how much I had, I sold him a pack of jumping jacks for seventy-five cents. Since I paid nothing for that pack, I made seventy-five cents straight profit. And it was right about here that the lightbulb went off.

I could sell these fireworks.

It would be really easy, too. I had more fireworks than I knew what to do with. I could keep them for personal use, but they were almost a burden. As I knew, my friends would constantly beg me for free packs, and the older kids would make sure that any cool fireworks I brought around the Park would be confiscated via wedgie. By selling them, I wouldn't have to deal with this and could make some money. And if I was selling them, the older kids wouldn't take them. Selling them was a way to legitimize the fact that I had them and portray myself as a businessman. The older kids could be dicks, but they weren't about to *rob* me.

Yes, I could sell these fireworks.

And I could make a lot of money.

After all, no one else sold fireworks. Or rather, no other eleven-year-old sold fireworks. Maybe some adults sold them, but they surely wouldn't sell them to kids, something I had no moral objection to doing, since *I* was a kid and all and these were my friends. One look at the jumping jacks or one thought of the potential destruction the firecrackers could cause and my friends would be desperate for more. How could they not be? And after that first taste, if they wanted more, they had to go through me, since I was the only game in town; without even realizing it, I had single-handedly cornered the market on illegal fireworks, with one bulk purchase from my supplier, Henry. I had the product, I was the only one with the product, and I was looking to liquefy.

Yes, I could sell these fireworks.

And yes, I could make a lot of money.

Holy crap.

But there was a problem: I was, for all intents and purposes, a shit dude. In the great social hierarchy of the neighborhood, while I wasn't at the bottom of the barrel, I certainly wasn't sitting at the top. I was not athletic, so I didn't garner popularity in that way. I had no older siblings or cousins, so no one my age outside of my friends knew my name or my family. And I was a model student, getting good grades and never causing any trouble at school, so I wasn't what teachers would call a "bad seed," which was a surefire way to gain notoriety in the neighborhood. Thinking about this in terms of a business plan, I knew I had friends whom I could sell to, but outside my circle of a dozen friends and another dozen acquaintances, I was unknown. If I wanted my new business to be successful, I would need more costumers than just my closest friends. And I wasn't popular enough to pull this off. I also figured that this illegal selling of fireworks would be hard work. My dad had bought me a lot of fireworks, and I would need help moving all of it. I *could* do it alone, but it would take up all my free time, time I needed for video games and listening to Guns N' Roses, Bobby Brown, and Tone Loc.* In short, I needed to take on a partner. And so I turned to my best friend David.

David is one of my oldest friends. Whenever we go drinking together today, if our level of intoxication is firmly in the "beer-soaked nostalgia" zone, we reminisce about his birthday party in first grade when I bought him a Big John Studd WWF wrestling figure—one of the thick rubber ones that I was immediately reminded of many years later when, for the first time, I stuck a dildo into a stripper at a friend's bachelor party—when he already had one, committing my first of many future party fouls. Back then, David was a small kid with giant ears but with street smarts to rival the older kids. Though we were both similar in our ability to BS people, David had a significant advantage where I didn't: older relatives. He had an older sister who hung around with the "older heads" (guys a few years older than us), as well as an older cousin who was a tough dude. Therefore David had immunity from getting picked on. Add in the fact that he played basketball very well and was known on many corners of Second Street because of this, and the choice was easy.

David was, in essence, the ideal partner for this business venture. Since he was small, quick, well-known, and well protected, he would be the runner/front man for the operation. The face of the business, he'd take care of the grunt work, being

---

* I had, and still have, rather eclectic tastes in music.

out on the street, taking orders, getting paid, driving his bike around with a backpack full of fireworks at all times. I, on the other hand, would be the Kingpin. Since I was larger, slower, less well-known, and much less protected, I would be the brains behind the operation. It would be my job to work the books, keeping track of all the orders and monies, while running the show from behind the curtain. The other reason this role was suitable to me was that should anything "go down," David would be the one taking the fall. I could easily get rid of notebooks that kept the names and corners of the customers. I could also get rid of the stash of fireworks that was hidden most excellently under my bed. If anything were to happen, I would get away scot-free, unless David ratted me out, which of course he would never do.*

We divided the partnership 75-25. The reason for the imbalance was simple: he needed me much more than I needed him. And there was the whole matter of how my dad bought the fireworks. We were running on profits because of his money. But David, like myself, had an enterprising spirit and so didn't put up an argument, as he was interested only in getting involved in a scheme.**

In less than a week, we ran through the $60 worth of fireworks my dad had first bought and made an astounding $140. Since we spent nothing, that was $140 in pure profit, $35 to Da-

---

* I never told David that this was part of the reason why I offered him this partnership. So now I have to be fully prepared for a punch in the face the next time I see him. Hi, Dave. Sorry about that.

** And for the record, I think this was the first and last time David got the raw end of a deal.

vid and $105 to me. Make no mistake, $105 for an eleven-year-old is an ungodly shitload of money. I was, for all intents and purposes, fucking filthy rich. Once David and I started making money, just like our customers who were purchasing our fireworks, we were hooked. Having spending money, enough to buy whatever struck our fancy (mostly slices of pizza and sodas), meant that David and I became instantly cool. David had been popular before, but for me this taste of fame was new and tantalizing. I had gone from the nerd who had won the spelling bee and cried when he finished second in the geography bee to the Guy Behind the Guy, Mr. Fireworks himself, the one who was so cool that he dealt not with his buddies—that job belonged to David, my assistant—but presumably with the adults and/or gangsters who sold him the fireworks. Word spread like wildfire through the neighborhood that Mulgrew and Floody were selling fireworks, and soon David was driving his bike as far away as Second and Reed to sell to some friends of friends up there. Business was booming (pun entirely intended).

But there was a problem. We were out of the goods and needed more. This presented a major bump in the road. I knew I couldn't ask my dad to buy me more fireworks. The paying part was not the problem, since David and I now had money and were willing to invest it. It was my dad's permission that would be difficult to get. I could only manipulate the postdivorce guilt so much, and telling him that I already went through $60 worth of fireworks in a week and needed more might raise some suspicions.

I realized that I'd have to go straight to Henry. I didn't know much about Henry, but he seemed like a nice guy. And he seemed . . . trusting, good-hearted. The only other thing I knew about Henry was that he smoked like a goddamn chimney. I thought my dad was bad with his two-pack-a-day habit, but this guy made my father look like a fourteen-year-old girl catching a smoke after geometry class. This was all I had to work with on Henry as I devised a strategy to get more product to keep the business going.

Finally, I had it. The following Saturday, David would follow me up to my dad's street, when I knew my dad was at work. Henry would be sitting on his porch, smoking a cigarette, like he always did. I'd act like I was dropping off something at my dad's house, but stop by to say hello. I'd tell him also that I had bought him a gift to thank him for the fireworks, a pack of Marlboro Reds. Henry, softened by my act of generosity, would then not bat an eyelash when I asked if, since I was here and all, I might be able to buy some more fireworks.

I realize that it might seem odd for an eleven-year-old to be gifting a pack of cigarettes to a fifty-year-old man, but at the time I saw nothing wrong with it. My friends were just starting to smoke at my age and I had been buying cigarettes for my dad since I was old enough to walk to the store alone. So buying a pack of cigarettes for an older guy wasn't a big deal. Hell, every year for his birthday, from the age of eight until high school, I used to buy my dad a carton of cigarettes—until I realized that I was helping him to slowly kill himself and that was probably a bad thing.

David waited around the corner and I headed up the block where, sure enough, Henry was on the porch having a smoke. "Hey, Henry."

"Oh—hey, Jason." He sat up from his reclined position and put out his cigarette. My dad did the same thing whenever he greeted someone. He sat up, put out his cigarette, and said hello. Then Henry, like my dad did, immediately lit another one. Why didn't he just put the first down? Wasn't that wasteful? "What are you up to?"

"I was just gonna drop some stuff off at my dad's, but I'm glad I saw you." I reached into the brown bag I was carrying. "I brought you something to say thanks for the fireworks." I handed him the pack of Reds.

Henry smiled. "Well, ain't that nice. That's nice. I'll have to tell your father about that."

Crap. I hadn't prepared for that. My dad knowing that I was here would seriously ruin my plot. But it was too late to turn back now. If I stopped or stumbled, the whole plan would fall apart.

"I was wondering if I might be able to buy some fireworks." I was rattled—I didn't mean to blurt this out like I did. I didn't stand a chance of scoring now.

"Well, I don't know." Henry smoked a third of his newly lit cigarette in one drag. "Does your dad know about this?"

"Yeah, he knows." I figured, what's one more lie? "He's just working a lot and he's gonna be working a lot over the next couple of days, so I figured I'd ask you."

The moment of truth. Henry took another third-of-a-cigarette drag, smiled, and said, "C'mon in."

In moments, I was walking out of Henry's house with plastic bags full of fireworks. I met David around the corner, and we stuffed our backpacks before heading off to the neighborhood. Like two junkies, we ripped into the brick of jumping jacks and lit some on the way home, even though it was daytime, just to feel the magic. And the magic, it was good.

And once again, FM Enterprises, what we called our business using the initials of our last names, was up and running. A start-up, we only sold the basics: firecrackers, jumping jacks, bottle rockets, and Roman candles, keeping simple to build capital and maximize profit. The order I got from Henry was the same order that my dad had gotten. He was surprised that I had the cash to buy $64 worth of fireworks, but I told him that it was recently my birthday and this was part of my present. $64 bought us:

- One brick of firecrackers (40 packs) for $9
- One brick of jumping jacks (48 packs) for $13
- Twelve packs of bottle rockets for $7
- A case of Roman candles (24 packs of 6 candles each) for $35

Our wholesale costs per item were then as follows:

- One pack of firecrackers: 23¢
- One pack of jumping jacks: 27¢
- One pack of bottle rockets: 58¢
- One pack (of 6) Roman candles: $1.45

When we sold packs individually, we charged:

- Firecrackers: 50¢
- Jumping jacks: 75¢

- Bottle rockets: $1
- Roman candles: $3

It figures that it was this part of the business I loved, the nerdy side. Before embarking on selling the original load of fireworks, I had guesstimated the cost per item based on what I thought he had paid for them. After buying our own, I learned that I was right and the prices we set on the first batch of fireworks were correct and sound. Finally, all that stupid math had a practical purpose.*

With the second shipment of fireworks secured back at my house, David and I were overjoyed and went about gettin' that cash. Sales continued to be high, as David made hourly bike runs to and from my house, dropping off money and picking up more fireworks. I kept all the cash in a "safe," which was actually a broken jewelry box that I picked out of the trash. It didn't even have a lock on it, but I continued to call it a safe and be secretive about it to give David the impression that I knew what I was doing and I was a professional. Image is important in any new business venture.

As the money continued to come in, I started dreaming big. I figured that this would go on forever and David and I would be millionaires around sophomore year in high school. In the meantime, I was planning on going to Tower Records to buy every CD they had. In a month or so, I'd ask my mom about getting a cable line in my room, so I could get a TV—

---

* I am actually kind of getting an erection thinking about all this math. I really, really wish this were a joke.

"Jimmy's family was getting rid of one" would be my reason for the presence of the television, when in reality I was going to head to Sears up on Oregon Avenue to buy the sweetest TV they had. And of course, my Sega Genesis would be hooked up to that gorgeous television, which I would play for approximately six hours a day. Video games, music, a giant TV—this was the life.

Or it was going to be. I never physically sold fireworks—that was David's job. At first, we were selective about to whom we sold. We didn't want some idiot getting hurt or some moron getting caught and ratting us out to his parents. David would only sell to friends or friends of friends whom we could trust. But the lust for more money and power made us sloppy. And by "us," I mean David.

If you wanted fireworks, you had to order them from David. David would come to me and I'd fill the order. Then he'd go out only with that order, get paid, and come back and give me the cash for safekeeping. Whenever he went out on runs, David carried only the fireworks necessary to fulfill the order. In this way, if anything happened to David (that is, he got beat up or otherwise lost the fireworks or money), we'd only lose that particular order. We didn't just set up shop on a corner and offer fireworks for sale. We were a serious business, not a fucking lemonade stand.

On a Thursday afternoon, David came by my place to make a run. I gave him the stuff and off he went. I was expecting him back in a half hour, probably less. But when an hour had passed and he hadn't returned, I grew agitated. I set off on my bike to head to Second and Mifflin to the schoolyard where David made the deal, but there was no sign of him. I went around the Park and couldn't find him there. I drove by his house and knocked. No answer. I went back to my house and waited. And waited. And waited some more. Nothing from David. But instead of going out again, I figured I'd stay in the house, in case he was trying to find me and we kept missing each other.

Around dinnertime, the phone rang.

"Hello?"

"You're lucky you answered the phone, boy, and not your mother."

It was David's mom, Eleanor.

"My son came home earlier today to get a Lunchable and guess what I found?"

"Um . . ."

"Let me tell you something," she said, on fire: "If I ever catch you and my son selling any more fireworks, I'll shove those fireworks right up your asses and light them! Do you understand?"

Fuck. "Yes."

"Now I'm not gonna tell your mother about this, because I know how upset she would be. But that's it. You got it?"

Fuck. "Yes."

"Good." She hung up.

Fuck.

A Lunchable, a Lunchable, my kingdom for a Lunchable.

And with that, FM Enterprises closed up shop. While I can't say that the remaining fireworks were destroyed, I can say that they were not sold. Mine and David's friendship remained strong, though to this day I don't understand why he couldn't have gotten the damn Lunchable *after* dropping off those fireworks. But then again, Lunchables are certainly delicious, so I can't blame him that much.

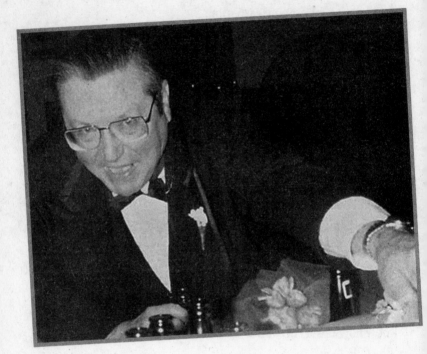

This is my grandpop.

And somewhere, my grandpop watched the rise and fall of my little empire, laughed, shook his head, and took a sip of his Manhattan. Jasper . . . so much to learn.

Chapter Seven

Uncle Petey

Uncle Petey moved to my block when I was eleven years old. He wasn't my uncle, but that's what I and all of my friends called him. I realize that anytime the moniker *uncle* is applied to a man, it conjures up all sorts of different images: an unshaven middle-aged man in a raggedy cardigan who promises you Skittles but instead gives you the ol' pat-down in his car; a *Sopranos*-esque goomba with tacky jewelry who yells a lot and strings together incoherent phrases like "bragadadooche!" and "madadeesh!"; a confirmed bachelor who shows up at holiday parties in neatly pressed clothes with his "roommate" Jonathan and uses adjectives like "delicious" and "gorgeous" while talking to your mom and the women in the family about a great new moisturizer he's using, while Uncle Joey and Uncle Eddie get into a shoving match in the living room over who was the better Eagles quarterback, Jaws or Randall.*

But Uncle Petey was none of these things. In many ways, he was your average nineteen-year-old kid. A little on the short side, with a slightly high-pitched voice and mousy features, he had an easy laugh and a thick South Philly accent. We called him Uncle Petey because he actually was the uncle of one of the kids I hung around with, my buddy Screech.** Screech would talk about how cool his Uncle Petey was so often that the name stuck in our circle of friends. We, even his own nephew, never called him "Uncle Petey" to his face, but rather only when referring to him in the third person. As a matter of fact, I'm sure that Petey would have been pretty weirded out if he knew we called him "Uncle Petey." What nineteen-year-old wants a gang of kids calling him "uncle"? I'm starting to feel a little uneasy even writing about it.

Petey was more like an older brother to us than anything else. A big part of being Irish Catholic is having an intense disdain for your siblings. I would guess that this disdain is directly inverse to the income of your household; the less money you have, the more you despise your siblings. One bathroom and two bedrooms between three or five or seven brothers and sisters isn't going to ease the tension any. Those of us who had

---

* With all due respect to the Polish Rifle, it's gotta be Randall.
** Screech got his own rather unoriginal nickname from the ubiquitous television show *Saved by the Bell* because he bore a slight resemblance, hairwise, to Dustin Diamond's nerdy character. Later in life, Screech's nickname would be changed to Nugget, for reasons unknown to me (and probably everyone else).

siblings were not close to them—especially at that age. We no longer viewed our brothers as friends, teammates, or partners in crime as we did earlier in life, but rather as potential foils, pains in the asses, and *Mommy said get out of the bathroom—I have to poop!*

But in Petey we found that older brother. It was only a matter of time after he moved onto the block that Screech would take us over to his place, where we could hang out in peace, without our parents or brothers and sisters bothering us. His house was an escape for us, where we could go to get out of our own homes, listen to music, and talk about things that interested us (especially sports and these fascinating things called "tits" that were starting to appear on the older girls). While we did most of this in the room that Screech claimed as his own, we hung out with Petey quite a lot, too. Petey was like us in many ways—a big kid who liked to play video games, curse, and break balls. But in other ways Petey was what we aspired to be: a man who knew about shit. To be a man who knew about shit or a man who knew shit was the neighborhood ideal, someone who was respected and who could dole out advice on any number of topics. Petey fit this profile. He knew a lot about sports. He knew (or claimed to know) a lot about women. And he knew a lot, a whole lot, about gambling.

Petey was a gambler. I'm not talking about cards or casinos here, but about sports. Pro and college football, baseball, pro and college basketball—hell, even figure skating, swimming, and gymnastics—there wasn't much Petey wouldn't bet on. Normally, this type of behavior could land a man in a lot of trouble. After college, I spent several years working in homeless shelters throughout the Northeast,* and many of the sad stories of the shelters' residents started with gambling problems. But Petey was good at gambling. Nay, Petey was *sublime*. Gambling, he'd tell us time and time again, was not about luck. It was about science. And Petey was a scientist par excellence.

Petey was also a bookie. For a percentage of the winnings, Petey took bets for someone. Petey was the neighborhood point man for that someone, taking bets over the phone and in person from guys in our area. Each week, Petey would collect and account for the all bets and money that he had handled during the week and pass this on to that someone. That someone might pass them on to someone else, who would then pass them on to someone else, all the way up the line to I-don't-know-what. I'd rather not think about that and I'd certainly rather not explore this here, lest I wake up in the morning with "Slow your roll, fat chops" painted in pig's blood on the door to my apartment. So let's just leave it alone for now.

Excellent gambler/bookie was an entirely acceptable profession in my neighborhood. It was even looked upon admirably. Nobody I knew grew up to be a doctor or a pilot or an inventor or anything cool like that. Once you graduated from high school, the laws of the neighborhood dictated that your career

---

*This is a complete lie, written to impress any attractive women reading. I never worked in any homeless shelter and don't know about any homeless people's stories. My editor made me put in this footnote explaining the truth—something about "not being irresponsible" or something. My only hope is that this footnote is so small that those attractive women reading the book don't read it. Keep your fingers crossed.

choices consisted of longshoreman, electrician, mechanic, roofer, or something similar. Each is a worthy profession in its own right, but not exactly what us kids aspired to be. If you could spend all day taking bets, studying sports, and yelling at horses, well, that's not a bad gig at all. It sure beats tarring a roof on a hot summer day or driving a forklift on a pier in windchills hovering around zero.

Being a gambler also gave you a certain neighborhood cache, for two reasons. One, it's a social profession. It requires you to be friend, confidant, and consoler to many people. Because Petey wasn't running the operation himself, he was never the bad guy. He was just taking the bets for someone else. He commiserated with those who lost, because he knew that feeling, too (although in most cases, considerably less than they did). Because he was so affable, he developed friendships with those from whom he took bets. And like your local dry cleaner, dentist, or barber, his business grew from referrals. Word of his charisma spread and eventually he was handling many, many bets, which in turn meant greater neighborhood "fame." Second, Petey made a lot of money doing what he did. And in a working-class neighborhood, few things garner respect or power the way that money—spent properly—does. Money was a tricky thing. If you spent it on extravagant things like nice cars or jewelry or big fur coats, you would be ostracized, called arrogant, and branded with the worst insult of all: someone who forgot where he came from (possibly because you dress like a pimp). Petey didn't wear jewelry or furs or drive around in a brand-new Cadillac; he had "The Bull," a mid-'80s Chevy Nova with peeling black paint and a "plush" red interior. By being down-to-earth and not living a garish lifestyle befitting a successful gambler and bookie, Petey showed us that it's okay to have money, but you have to spend it wisely.

But that doesn't mean you couldn't have fun with it. After all, what good is money if it can't provide at least a small measure of happiness? And what is fun if it's not taking your nephew's twelve-year-old friend to play video games against grown Puerto Rican men for obscene sums of money? What about using money as bait to watch some kids and buddies try to eat one of the hottest peppers on earth? That's fun, right?

As I mentioned, one of the main things we did at Uncle Petey's house was play video games. We often escaped to Petey's to get out of our houses, and since he didn't work, he was home all the time just hanging out. Screech would bring us over and we'd spend hours in front of one of the two TVs in Petey's living room, battling each other while Petey made calls, wrote down bets, or yelled at whatever player was fucking up his over/under bet by missing open layups.

This was the early '90s, before the souped-up video games that are on the market now. These were the days when sixteen-bit graphics were groundbreaking, when Nintendo was just about to give way to Sega Genesis, and before John Madden had figured out how to make himself (even more of) a multimillionaire by lending his likeness and voice to a video game. We weren't able to amuse ourselves with punching hookers in the latest Grand Theft Auto incarnation, so we had to stick to the basics. Mario was still King. And Luigi, well, he was always kind of off, right?

As a kid, I was a video game god. It may sound like I'm bragging here, but this is a statement of fact, pure and simple. You're probably surprised at this revelation: an unathletic smart kid, good at video games. Shocking, I know. Though I couldn't field a fly ball or make a layup, I could do some serious damage in RBI Baseball and I would take you to school in Double Dribble. Not only that, I could conquer the nonsports games as well. Give me a rainy Saturday morning and I would have Link and Princess Zelda kissing by dinnertime. While you might gape when after beating Metroid for the first time you learned that *he* was actually a *she*, this wouldn't surprise me, since I beat the game before you (and once last week, too).

This continued into my preteen years, but by then I had dropped the other types of games and stuck only to the sports games, where I really made my mark. I imagined that I played these games with such fervor and would savor each victory so intensely precisely because I was—to put it mildly— the worst athlete in the history of the world. In the video game realm, I found my calling and my escape. What I could not achieve in reality, I could achieve in virtual reality. In Nintendo or Sega Genesis, I could hit eight three-pointers in a half or grab the winning touchdown and do it with grace and aplomb, visions of camera bulbs flashing in my head and snippets of my postgame interviews replaying on all the local newscasts. In this way I could prove to my friends that I was worthy of respect, an athlete in my own way and a force to be

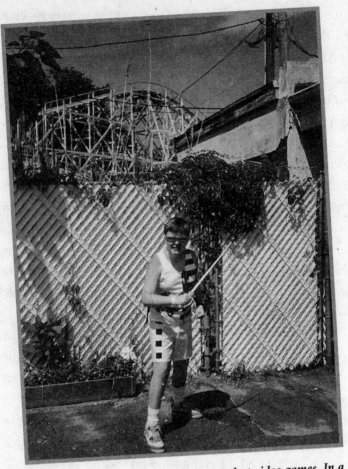

Believe it or not, this kid was really good at video games. In a related story, he would not lose his virginity until he was almost twenty years old.

reckoned with. But like many superior athletes, my incredible prowess went straight to my head. It wasn't long before I became unbearable to play against, as I ran up scores, taunted opponents during the games, and gloated after victories. And it wasn't long before Petey picked up on my abilities and decided he could make some cash off them.

South Philly as we knew it was very segregated. The Irish Americans lived on the south end of Second Street and the streets surrounding it; Polish Americans were scattered just north of the Irish Americans; the Asians—a mix of Cambodians, Koreans, and Vietnamese—lived above Fifth Street; the blacks were just north of them. But nestled in the middle of the Irish neighborhood was one street, a single street, full of Puerto Rican families. The non–Puerto Ricans in the area were unsure how this street came to exist, but it developed into its own small community (read: it had a grocery store and a bar, really the only two necessities in our neighborhood). Though whitey was not discouraged from walking along this street, it was usually avoided if possible. Petey, on the other hand, dealt with and knew all the Puerto Ricans, as gambling knows no race, creed, gender, and, um, however the rest of that line goes. More important, Petey knew how seriously they took their video games, often having daylong tournaments, betting on games, and partying.

The way Petey explained it, it would be very simple. He and I would head down to Little Puerto Rico, I'd play a couple of video games against the guys there at his friend Ricky's house, I'd win, and I'd get some money. "'Cause you'll win, right?" Petey asked. Yes, I said, but I was too dumbfounded to say anything else. Besides, we were already outside Ricky's house by the time Petey told me of this plan, so I didn't have much of a choice.

The preferred game in Little Puerto Rico was Sega's newly released NHLPA Hockey '93,* the revolutionary game that would spawn annual incarnations over the next dozen-plus years. This game was eons better than Nintendo's Ice Hockey, which had previously been *the* hockey video game, famous for allowing the game player to pick his or her combination of fat player/medium player/thin player in his line. Nowadays, video games are so advanced that consumers are hard pressed to be truly blown away by any single release (the only recent exception I can think of is the aforementioned Grand Theft Auto series). But NHLPA Hockey '93 introduced actual NHL teams and players, with much better graphics and increased maneuverability. When it was released, it truly was a watershed moment for video game enthusiasts like myself, probably the greatest day of my life to that point.**

I won't get into the irony of a bunch of Puerto Ricans playing and loving a hockey video game—that's like my white friends and I getting really into a video game called Prison Yard: Fight for Survival—but they were very serious about it. Petey and I entered Ricky's house as two guys were playing Hockey '93, and to a chubby twelve-year-old white kid

---

* Which EA Sports actually released in 1992, one year before I graduated eighth grade.

** Cut me some slack—I wouldn't touch a boobie until about four years later, so I had to take joy in other, less boobilicious moments. (Okay, seven years later. And it was my own. Don't be a dick about it.)

like myself, it was an intimidating scene. Hell, to a chubby twenty-nine-year-old white guy it would be an intimidating scene. Since it was summer, every guy in the house had his shirt off, showing off both his flashy gold chains and his tattoos, the latter of which could be divided into two categories: a) female names or b) Jesus. The room was cloudy with smoke, a little tobacco, a little pot. Everybody was drinking beer while watching the two players on the Sega Genesis. I stood quietly next to Petey. No one even noticed I was there. If they did, they certainly didn't question it.

I was introduced to Ricky, the proprietor of the establishment. Ricky had a broad, welcoming smile and fingers the size of sausage links. With his easygoing manner, he could have been nicknamed "The Mayor." What was different about Ricky was that unlike the rest of the Puerto Ricans, he was wearing a shirt, probably because he was ginormously fat. For this reason I liked him—I was afraid that it might be a house rule that everyone had to take their shirt off. But despite our chubby kinship and his friendliness, I still wanted to get the hell out of there as quickly as possible.

Ricky turned to Petey after saying hello to me and the two of them started talking gambling shop. I watched the two guys playing Hockey '93 to see what they were all about. Like real sports, in sports video games you can gather what an opponent is capable of doing, his inclinations, his strengths, and his weaknesses, by watching him. Truth be told, both of these guys sucked. Though one was beating the other handily, they both played the same way—selfishly. They kept going for the big check or the big breakaway goal, never passing the puck. Though five guys per team were on the ice, it was like a constant game of one-on-one. Screech, Jimmy, and Chuckie played this way, too. Sports video games lend themselves to this type of play. They are primarily exercises in role playing, as the user pretends to be the star of the team. In the name of glory, sound play is compromised for the exciting goal, the long touchdown pass, or the high-flying dunk. But while this type of play is certainly entertaining, it doesn't always lead to a victory.

In no other sports video game is sound play more abandoned than in hockey. This is understandable, since there's not much cooler in the video game realm then scoring a goal on a breakaway or crushing your opponent with a monster check against the boards. But a seasoned video game vet like me knew this type of play was flawed and very easy to exploit. Above all else, patience is key in hockey, and I used my patience and their lack of it to my advantage. While an opponent would recklessly send player after player at me, I would try to move the puck around as quickly as possible. All the movement on his team's behalf would eventually create an open shooting lane and then—bam! That's when I would unleash a one-timer, a shot made in hockey just as the pass from a teammate arrives in front of you.* If done properly, it rarely fails

---

* A better example: Player 1 and Player 2 are on the same team. Player 1 skates along the boards toward the net, Player 2 straggles behind. When a passing lane opens up, Player 1 passes the puck back or across the ice to Player 2, whose stick is already raised, cocked for the shot and ready to go. When the puck arrives in front of Player 2, he shoots. Because the shooter's stick was already raised and he did not need to wind up, the goalie has less time to prepare and set himself for the shot. The result? GGGGGOOOOOAAAAALLLLLL!!!!!!

to score a goal in video games. And you can bet that I almost always did it properly.

Even though I knew their style of play, since my friends played the same way, I was nervous as I sat down to start. I drew Francisco (called Franky), the victor of the game I had watched. Franky was wearing a loose-fitting tank top, exposing his muscles, which were not insignificant. I sat to his left and could see that his left pec read like a scroll of papyrus, listing names of people, men and women, who I presumed were close to his heart. Despite this seemingly sensitive body art, Franky was a total dick to me. I'm not sure why a twenty-year-old shirtless Puerto Rican guy would feel the need to talk shit to a kid, but he started into me as soon as I sat down. My favorite of his barbs was that since I wasn't "jacked" (muscular), I would suck at the game. Because scientists have long noted the correlation between physical fitness and video game ability. Fucking asshole.

But I didn't listen to his chatter and it was extra special for me when I had the opportunity to embarrass him in front of his friends, running up goal after goal as Petey screamed in the background, "I told you! I told you!" I don't remember much of the game; it was just a beating, plain and simple. Franky's buddies started breaking his balls about how he was getting busted up by a kid, and they were cheering me on, calling for more blood, as the familiar sound of the goal siren blared from the television. At the end of the game, Franky sulked away without looking back at me. After I won that game, I played another. My next opponent was much nicer and didn't talk shit to me, but I still dispatched him easily. All told I played four games, going 4-0. *Cómo hace ese gusto,* bitches?

While this was arguably the greatest athletic achievement of my life, Petey was also having a ball, laughing it up each time I scored and after each victory. I'm not sure what he enjoyed more about that night, that I was winning or that he was making money. He had made a series of bets on the games and was raking in the cash after each win. I don't know how much he won that evening, but I did get a cut of the winnings, a nice fat twenty-dollar bill. And I mean this sincerely. Twenty dollars for playing four video games was not a bad day's work for me, almost a week's salary delivering papers. I could get used to this.

But before I had to concern myself with reporting this new income stream to the IRS, our arrangement fell apart. I only returned to Little Puerto Rico two more times, getting twenty bucks for each visit. Prior to entering Ricky's house the second time, Petey pulled me aside and gave me a little pep talk. "I want you to really beat the fuck out of them. Score as many goals as you can." I guess the spreads were increasing with each victory. The results were the same on both return trips: big victories. After the third visit, I was in Petey's house and asked him when we'd be heading back to Little Puerto Rico. He said, "Nah, we ain't going back no more," adding, "But good job . . . jerk-off" and handing me another twenty.

That was as close to a seal of approval that one could get from Petey and I happily accepted it. I put the money in my pocket and headed up to Screech's room to discuss the news of the day. I was feeling down that our little adventure was over, but I knew it was only a matter of time before another came along.

* * *

The Scotch bonnet pepper is native to Jamaica and Belize. The pepper, which is about the size and shape of a below-average adult male's tightened scrotum, changes colors as it ripens, going from green to yellow to orange to red. But don't let its funny shape and pretty colors fool you—it is a badass motherfucker.

What makes a pepper hot is the amount of capsaicin it contains. Capsaicin is the nasty lil' chemical that makes you feel like your lips, tongue, and mouth are on fire when you have that first "nuclear" buffalo wing. While most people rely on the counter girl at their local chicken place or the big board hanging behind her when deciding on how hot they want their wings (mild–medium–hot–nuclear–the universe collapses onto itself and life ceases to exist for the remainder of eternity, etc.), there exists a scientific construct used to measure the heat of peppers: the Scoville scale. According to Wikipedia*:

> *[The Scoville scale] is named after Wilbur Scoville, who developed the Scoville Organoleptic Test in 1912. As originally devised, a solution of the pepper extract is diluted in sugar water until the "heat" is no longer detectable to a panel of (usually five) tasters; the degree of dilution gives its measure on the Scoville scale. Thus a sweet pepper, containing no capsaicin at all, has a Scoville rating of zero, meaning no heat detectable even undiluted.*

---

* Sorry, but Wikipedia is just about the extent of my researching prowess. And no, I don't care that I'm not putting my history degree to good use.

An example to help explain. Your typical jalapeño is in the bottom third of the Scoville ladder, coming in at 2,500 to 8,000 units. As Wikipedia points out, that means that its extract has to be diluted 2,500–8,000-fold before the capsaicin, the heat of the pepper, can no longer be tasted. Conversely, our friend the Scotch bonnet is near the top of the Scoville ladder, measuring anywhere between 100,000 and 325,000 Scoville units. Therefore, it needs to be diluted up to 325,000-fold before you can't feel its heat. That's some serious fire.*

How a case of these peppers ended up in Petey's hands is unknown. One could buy them at a gourmet grocery store, but there were no gourmet grocery stores on Second Street. And I don't think Petey grabbed some on a trip into Center City, Philadelphia's downtown, while picking up the ingredients for his famous red wine reduction, since I never saw Petey actually make anything, although once I did see him microwave a pack of cigarettes when he was drunk after an Eagles game. Most likely, some came in "through longshore." This means that a ship carrying the peppers docked on a port on the Delaware River. I can see it now: a produce ship from South America (or wherever the hell Belize is) comes in and the crew tells the local longshoremen about the legend of Scotch bonnet, *La Pimienta del Diablo*. After getting a complimentary case of the

---

* In Scoville units, there is only one pepper hotter than the Scotch bonnet: the Red Savina habañero. According to redsavina.com, just one gram of the Red Savina can cause detectable heat in 1,272 pounds of sauce, which is roughly equivalent to the amount my Uncle John consumes every two years. The only thing hotter than the Red Savina that is not a derivation of the capsaicin chemical compound is pepper spray. That's right, mace. This stuff is not for the uninitiated.

peppers,* one neighborhood guy thinks to himself, "I know a guy who'd have some fun with these . . ." And once Petey got a hold of the Scotch bonnets, in his infinite mischievous wisdom he devised a contest. The word quickly spread through the neighborhood. Anyone who could eat the peppers and go an allotted time (thirty seconds, sixty seconds, etc.) without drinking anything would get cash. Simple as that.

This was one of the first times that I doubted Petey. I didn't see what he had to gain in this experiment, so I didn't know why he would make this offer. I figured that obviously someone, probably several people, could eat this pepper with ease. Not me—I still brushed my teeth with bubble gum–flavored toothpaste because I thought that the mint variety was too spicy, and the very smell of buffalo wings would send me hiding to my room until the house was properly fumigated—but a lot of people liked peppers. And as for those who didn't win the bet and had to drink the water, so what? It's too hot, they drink the water, they cool off, and that's it. What's so great about that? Of course, neither I nor anyone else knew about the strength of these peppers. To us, they were just glorified jalapeños, a minor obstacle in the way of making a quick fifty dollars. Uncle Petey would have the last laugh.

My call came on a summer evening with a knock at the door. This was early on in the contest, perhaps even the second day. I hadn't heard of anyone who had actually tried to eat the pepper yet, and I was only vaguely interested. My indifference stemmed from my aforementioned confusion as to why Petey

---

* Read: "After stealing a case of the peppers."

would have the contest in the first place. My friends Jimmy (called "the Muppet," because he was small and looked like a Muppet) and Chuckie (nicknamed "Eclipse," because he was big and blocked out the sun) were on my porch trying to convince me to come up to Petey's house to try the pepper. In my most diplomatic way, I vehemently objected to any participation in such a contest, citing my lack of tolerance for any and all spice. Before I could properly launch into my spiel about how the whole thing was stupid anyway, Chuckie reached into his pocket and pulled out a fifty-dollar bill. He looked smugly at me and said, "I did it." Knowing that fifty dollars was enough to get me by for a solid month, I looked at Jimmy, shocked, and he added, "I *almost* did it. I got to twenty-eight seconds, but had to take a drink. And Petey wouldn't give me nothing." My eyes drifted back to the fifty that Chuckie held in front of him, and my mind was made up even before he said, "Seriously, you should try it."

Down to Petey's I marched, followed by Eclipse and the Muppet, where I found Petey and Screech waiting for me. Like a chubby, sexually insecure mouse being led to a trap, they even had one of the bonnets out and a glass of water on the end table next to the couch, ready to go. Petey sat in his recliner, looking intently and trying to hide a mischievous smile, at that moment looking very much the part of Rat Bastard. I was ready for my cheese, thank you.

I was sat down on the couch and was debriefed. Eat the pepper and go thirty seconds without drinking the water and I get fifty dollars. Go a whole minute and I get a hundred. As Petey went over the rules, Jimmy the Muppet again lamented, "Man, I can't believe I missed it by two seconds!"

Petey gave me the pepper and I looked it over. It was small and green and looked unimposing. I decided that my best recourse would be to put the whole pepper in my mouth, chew it up, and swallow it down, rather than nibble away at it. I looked at the guys and told them I was ready, and Petey put on the TV Guide channel, which had the time in seconds and would act as a stopwatch for the event. When the clock struck exactly 7:12 P.M., I popped the pepper into my mouth. It had begun.

For about two seconds, I thought I was going to walk out with a hundred dollars in cash. The texture of the skin of the Scotch bonnet was sturdy but slightly chewy, the inside mostly hollow and a little moist. As my teeth clenched over the skin and began to mash the pepper, I felt very little heat at all, and heard just the crunch under my teeth. *I can do this*, I thought. *I can definitely do this*.

But then the inside of the pepper, with its moist inner walls covered in small seeds, reached my gums. And the underside of my tongue. And the inside of my cheeks.

And then my mouth completely exploded.

Each little seed, of which there were dozens, expended and injected an enormous amount of heat into my mouth and my body. Each one was like a land mine, like a land mine on cocaine, and all these coked-up land mines were spreading around my mouth, lodging themselves into the fleshy insides of my cheeks, between my teeth, burrowing into the recesses in the very top and in the very bottom of gums and where my teeth and gums met, exploding with a heat I never dreamed could exist in food form; such heat should be reserved only for weapons of destruction and celestial beings. My mouth was stinging sharply and my breathing became slow and heavy, each breath like I was shooting fire from my mouth and nostrils. The pain was overwhelming in the most literal sense; I could not process the trauma that was going on and all reason escaped me—what was happening to me allowed no room for thought and my body was reacting on its own, without any help or direction from me. I lost control of all the bodily fluids of my face: Tears were streaming from my eyes, drool from my mouth, and snot from my nose. Every pore of skin on my body opened up and sweat surged out. I could feel it coming out of my armpits, covering my forehead, in the small of my back, on my thighs, and even in my feet. I began to shake. I swallowed the pepper (or rather, the pepper slid down my throat) and I could feel it being swept past my tonsils and down my esophagus into my stomach like a heat-seeking missile.

I stumbled off the couch and from my knees reached for the water, which I poured down my throat, doing so with such urgency that I spilled it over my mouth and shirt. The pepper's seeds had successfully turned my saliva into hot lava, a thick, mucusy acidic potion, a condition made worse by the introduction of the water. Before, the pain was somewhat localized, restricted to my mouth and the back of my throat. Drinking the water was like pouring kerosene on a kitchen fire, and now the pain extended to my whole esophagus, my lips, and even my face. Now the whole house was on fire.

I looked up and through the tears I could see my four "friends"—Petey, Screech, Jimmy, and Chuckie—doubled over in laughter at my condition, their eyes also filled with tears (albeit for a very different reason). I decided that I would torture and murder them at a later date, but at the moment I was more concerned with putting an end to this pain that I was certain was going to kill me. I made a decision. Since there was no way I was going to be able to deal with this heat, this pepper had to come out. I ran or stumbled or clawed my way upstairs to the bathroom followed by the four idiots. I fell to its warm tile floor, made sticky by the summer heat and humidity, and kneeled over the toilet. I tried to make myself vomit, but this plan back-fired. The heat of the pepper mixed with my stomach acid was an unholy concoction and it was when I felt it rise from my belly into my throat that I began to scream (or yelp or whine). Puking is nasty enough in itself, and trying to make yourself puke is even worse. But the pain of inducing vomit after consuming one of the world's hottest peppers is a displeasure that I would not wish on any other human being, no matter how full of rage I may become.

Petey, Screech, Jimmy, and Chuckie were still in hysterics, crowding around the bathroom door, their heads poking around the edges of the door frame, watching me retch on the floor. I heaved again and again, choking back the bile and pepper juice, nearly suffocating from the heat. I couldn't throw up, I couldn't get the heat to stop, I was stuck. Broken and defeated, I lay there on the bathroom floor, swallowing back vomit and drinking water straight from the spigot of the bathroom faucet, desperate but with nowhere else to turn, waiting for the heat to just go away. Seconds or minutes or hours passed there on the floor: me unsuccessfully and involuntarily heaving into the toilet, me kneeling to drink water from the sink, repeat. When it stopped being interesting, the guys retreated back downstairs. The show was over for them. The pricks.

Eventually—and I use that word in the broadest possible sense—I started to regain control of my body. I was able to walk down the stairs, still shaky, where once again I was greeted by the laughter of my friends. Petey came up to me as I reached the bottom of the stairs, slapped me on the back with one hand while he wiped the tears from his face with the other, and said, "That was the best one yet!"

Then it was confession time. It turned out that Screech, Jimmy, and Chuckie had all faced similar fates as I had. None was able to successfully eat the Scotch bonnet and win the cash and all had equally miserable experiences. The key was information control. Screech, as he was Petey's nephew, was the first to try the pepper, in the presence of only Petey and a couple of his buddies. After he had failed spectacularly, crying and screaming at Petey for more water, he was "in." Screech then duped Jimmy into trying the pepper the same way that I was duped: by showing up at his house with the fifty-dollar bill, telling him that if he could do it, anyone could. Jimmy fell for it. Then Jimmy and Screech did the same to Chuckie. And Chuckie fell for it. And so it went with me. I too was now in on the joke, and that proved to be the only silver lining from the whole experience. Over the next couple of days, I watched countless people try the peppers, and these were some of the most memorable and funniest days of my life.* Everyone from the neighborhood came in to try the pepper, from kids my age to Petey's friends and even some fathers, and I was one of the select few who got to watch each sad attempt. Watching a person trip or seeing a man get hit in the balls has always been the gold standard, but I'd like to introduce a new contender to the physical comedy throne: watching someone eat a superhot pepper and almost die in a pool of their own sweat, drool, snot, and tears. If you haven't seen this, I feel sorry for you.

The peppers eventually ran out, or people wised up and stopped competing; I'm not sure which. After the peppers, Petey cemented his legacy as the neighborhood prankster. Individuals would go on to tell of their horrifying experiences with the peppers, at bars, at their jobs, to their friends and families, and Petey was at the center of every story. Those who tried and failed could only shake their head at the end of their tale and say, "That motherfucker Petey Duffy," with more than a tinge of respect, and maybe even a hint of affection.

That was Petey's gift: his levity. I suppose I could dig deeper and write about how, in his own twisted way, he taught us about male bonding, and by extension about humility, by taking us down a notch or two when we thought we were hot shit, and confidence, by praising us and treating us like his friends and equals, not some kids who hung out with his nephew. But Petey

---

* That is, once my mouth and face stopped hurting and I got my senses of smell and taste back. I am forever indebted to my mother, who, after smacking me around for being such a moron, put me on a steady diet of white bread and vanilla ice cream to get rid of the heat. I am still on this diet today, though not for pepper-related reasons.

would have none of that. He'd say that was a ballbuster, plain and simple, and we were his targets. And that's fine, because in some ways that's true. But I know that he would ask, like he always asked, "It was fun, right?" And me and Screech and Jimmy and Chuckie and everyone else would have to say, "Fucking-A right, it was."

Now if there was only a way for us to get *him* to eat that pepper.

Post Script

I have told what is now known as "The Uncle Petey Pepper Story" dozens—possibly hundreds—of times since it happened in the early '90s. And every time I finish telling it, I'm met with the same reaction: "Dude, you're a pussy. I love hot food—I could totally eat that pepper."* Obviously, this is something easier said than done, and each time I faced this retort I only strengthened my resolve that the next time I told the story I'd be sure to carry a Scotch bonnet, just to whip it out in front of the nonbeliever to say, "Yeah, well, try it, bitch." Unfortunately, my amazing capacity for laziness far surpasses my desire for vengeance, so I never grew motivated enough to actually go to the fancy grocery store to buy the pepper for my glorious retort.

A year after I graduated from college, I was living in New York City working as a paralegal at a large corporate law firm.

---

* You're probably saying this right now, ain't ya?

Over happy-hour drinks, I told the Uncle Petey Pepper Story to some friends and coworkers. They turned out to be much more ambitious than I was, and we were shortly planning our own Pepper Party. The concept was simple: the fifteen dollars it costs to get into our little shindig would cover the cost of booze and the prize money. Just because you came to the party, you did not have to eat the pepper—that was optional. We would have a sign-up sheet, and unlike Petey's contest, there would be no time markers for cash awards. We thought this would get too complicated so instead we decided that all contestants would eat the peppers at the same time. The last one standing who didn't drink or eat anything would get the cash. The rest of the party would cry tears of laughter as contestants fell into parox-ysms of pain. A good time would be had by all.

We were able to get the Scotch bonnets from a Jamaican grocery store in Queens, grabbing a few dozen of the little bas-tards. I had not seen the peppers since that summer at Petey's house, and when I looked at them in their little plastic bags, I got chills. Or rather, I should say, sweats. After the incident, I looked at the Scotch bonnets in the same way that I imagine a shark attack victim thinks of sharks, postattack—with an unnerving sense of terror but also a profound sense of respect. I daresay that there was also a sense of kinship, as if I could approach the bonnets and say offhandedly, "So, how about these poor bastards? They have no idea what they're getting into, the stupid sons of bitches!" And the peppers and I would laugh, laugh, and laugh, and maybe go grab a drink and catch a game.

In addition to the peppers, we also made sure to get lots of booze, some liquid courage to help any takers on the action. We didn't know how many people would be willing to eat the peppers, and so we also got lots of white bread, milk, and ice cream. This way we could ensure successful triage if needed, coaxing those who weren't 100 percent sure into taking the chance. Every contestant had heard the story, but none had previously eaten the pepper. This didn't stop the contestants from displaying various level of arrogance running the gamut from "I'm pretty sure I can do this" to "You might have to give me two." But as you might guess, they weren't feeling so full of themselves once they popped the bonnet. One thing that was different this time around was the availability and consumption of booze, an unfortunate upshot (no pun intended) of which was that people were throwing up everywhere (though we had large trash cans set up for such purposes). It went from funny to really funny to nasty to oh-man-that's-terrible very, very quickly.

And there was another difference this time around. Someone ate the pepper without a problem. A guy named Calvin, who said his parents raised him on a steady diet of spicy foods, ate the pepper and stood calmly as the people around him descended into hysterical madness. While water and milk were spilling everywhere, people were vomiting into the trash cans, and slices of white bread were flying through the air, Calvin chewed his pepper, swallowed it, and sat back and waited to be named the winner. He was cold as *ice*, and we could only assume that he spent a portion of his childhood living on a pepper farm and/or the sun.

So the moral of the story is that yes, it can be done. But at

the same time, please *do not try this at home*. I don't want to
be held responsible for anyone getting seriously hurt because
they tried to eat a hot pepper, and if you have a heart condition
or high blood pressure, you may actually die if you attempt
to do this.* Not because I have a conscience or anything, but
because I already have enough legal problems on my hands.
Thank you for your understanding and cooperation.

---

* My blood pressure is the reason that I did not eat a pepper at the Pepper
Party or in preparation for writing this book. I earned my stripes and did it
once, which is about four times too many.

Chapter Eight

Intermezzo: The Top Six Most Influential Songs of My Adolescence

"Crazy for You" Madonna

If you were to stop a person on the street and ask him or her what lovemaking sounds like, he or she might moan, shout, purr, or, in the case of my ex-girlfriend, make absolutely no sound except for saying, "Seriously, you're not done yet?" after about forty seconds. If I were one of the people you stopped and you asked me what lovemaking sounds like, I'd take off my

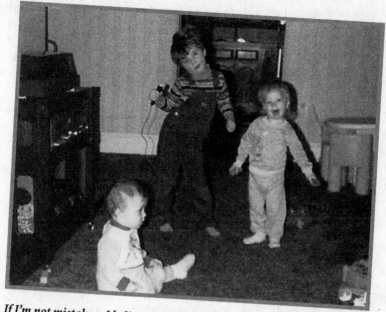

If I'm not mistaken, I believe I was reprising John Travolta's Danny Zuko in this photo.

iPod, put it on your ears, then play this song. Then you and I would make love. Not right there on the street, but in my car, which is parked right around the corner. It's not far, I swear.

I did not know what the word *sensual* meant when I first heard this song as a seven-year-old, but last year when I finally did learn what it meant, I immediately thought of "Crazy for You." While Madonna has been known as the embodiment of sexuality throughout her career, in this song she expresses a more delicate and vulnerable side of herself and her music. This is what makes this song unique and all the more appealing. While "Like a Virgin" is a thinly veiled satire that overflows with sexuality, "Crazy for You" oozes with genuine naïveté. At first, the protagonist appears to be cool and confident in a sexual setting (the dance floor), but soon she reveals her anxiousness and unfamiliarity with her simple, poignant lyrics ("I never wanted anyone like this . . .", "Trying hard to control my heart . . .", "It's so brand-new . . .", etc.).

But any way that I analyze it, one fact remains constant: this song gets me hot. To this day, I have an unhealthy obsession with it. Every time I hear it I experience the same reaction—I feel nervous, I get sweaty, and then something comes out of my bird that is like pee but not quite because it's clearer and more sticky and it smells like bleach. If I ever found a woman with low enough self-esteem or one who spoke such poor English I could trick her into agreeing to it, I would make love while this song played, on a bed of red silk sheets, in a room filled with tall candles, with slow, open-mouthed kisses, fingers passionately running through hair, a bowl of strawberries and whipped cream on the bedside table, and me in a Dracula costume. Until that happens, I'll have to stick to the status quo—jacking off at work while this plays on my iPod. Let's hope that by next Valentine's Day I'll have a reason to buy the red silk sheets I've always wanted.

"Look Away" Chicago

In no point in the history of art, literature, or music has the essence of lost love been captured and analyzed with such grace, beauty, and sorrow as it has in this song. Neruda came close in his "Tonight I Can Write the Saddest Lines" and in his "Song of Despair"; the story of the ill-fated love between Héloïse and Abélard may stir similar emotions; the breakup of Ross and Rachel tugged at our collective heartstrings. But it was the prog-rock band Chicago and the songwriting genius of Diane Warren that taught yours truly about the depths and darkness of love.

In the song, the protagonist learns that his former lover, their relationship having been mutually ended only a short time before, has found a new lover. Devastation so enraptures him that he pleads, if they should see each other socially, that she "look away," lest she see his tears of regret.

[*pause*]

I'll give you a moment to collect yourself, what with your heart most likely having just exploded in your chest.

Why I related so intensely to this song, I don't know, but I did. True, I was ten years old when this song first hit the airwaves. And true, what I knew of love at the time was limited to Tastykakes and my hamster, Boojee. But hearing this song was like being awakened and guided by the heartfelt and pained vocals of Bill Champlain into a world in which love is master, cruel master. Other songs had taught me of the glory of love (like, for example, "The Glory of Love" by former Chicago singer Peter Cetera), but this was the first to introduce me to the other side of the coin, showing me the perilous yin to love's joyful yang. And while I still have yet to experience love—that's a pretty complete emotion for someone who broke up with his last girlfriend to start dating a sausage—I am still grateful to Ms. Warren and Chicago for warning me, at an early age, about the dangers of love and heartbreak. Without their introduction by way of "Look Away," I would surely be writing this from a mental institution.

"Can You Stand the Rain" New Edition

I can say with a great degree of certainty that I was one of the only straight white boys in the greater Philadelphia area who wanted more than anything else to be a member of New Edition. If there were others, I would like to meet them. Perhaps we can start some sort of club or something. That might be nice.

New Edition does not get proper treatment by music historians, falling as they did between the Jackson 5, with whom they shared race and an advanced degree of musicality, and the New Kids on the Block, with whom they shared producers and hometown. The Jackson 5 grew out of the Motown era and was the launching pad for one of the most successful careers in music history (and in general weirdness) in the person of Michael Jackson. The New Kids on the Block were an astoundingly successful group of marginally talented Massholes whose claim to fame was that they served as fodder for masturbatory fantasies for girls the world over before those girls even understood what the words *masturbatory* and *fantasy* meant. New Edition is now unfairly known as that group Bobby Brown was in before he grew up to be a crazy person and married Whitney Houston.

If there is one thing I would like to accomplish, it is to let the world know about the greatness of New Edition. However, that seems like a lot of work, so I'll just explain why I love this song and then head back to bed.

Playing on the universal and time-tested metaphor of rain as trouble, what the group is trying to determine in "Can You Stand the Rain" is if the woman or lover can handle the difficult times. It is a simple and effective theme that spoke to me on many levels as a nine-year-old, curious as I was about how my girlfriend and I would handle those difficult times in our relationship, most of which I assumed would revolve around why I was so reluctant to take my shirt off at the beach. But it is not so much the theme of the song that affected me, but the sheer beauty of the vocals.

While I was a fan of New Edition's earlier stuff with the aforementioned cantankerous Bobby Brown ("Mr. Telephone Man," "Candy Girl," "Popcorn Love," "Cool It Now," etc.), I preferred their more mature sound with Johnny Gill. This is not because I felt that Gill's songs were catchy or better written, but because of the incredible vocal talent of the man himself.

If you are unfamiliar with the voice of Johnny Gill, you are an incomplete person. His voice is a masterwork, like an orgasm covered in chocolate. From the start of this song, as soon as I hear his voice, I immediately know that I am safe, loved, and sexually adequate. The first time I heard Johnny sing this song, I felt alternatively blessed and saddened: blessed to hear such incredibly dulcet and ebonylicious tones; saddened because I knew that for the rest of my life my ears would be merely empty shells of cartilage, occupied only with nostalgia, possessed by longing, forever hoping to feel what they felt the first time they heard Johnny Gill so sweetly sing, "Tell me, can you weather a storm?" Put simply, if God had a voice, His voice would be shit compared to Johnny Gill's.

(But let's hope He's not black. Because if He is, I am in serious, serious trouble. I don't even want to think about this right now. Let's move on—quickly.)

It is for this reason that I include this song on my list. "Can You Stand the Rain" opened my life to a world of aural pleasure that was previously unimaginable. There are few songs in my life that I've been compelled to say "Wow" to after listening to them for the first time, and not only is this a member of that exclusive group, but it's also the founder and president. My very idea of music and its potential was changed because of this song. And all I can offer in return is a simple affirmative—yes, I can stand the rain. Not because I am a strong man, but because with this song, and with that voice, anything is possible.

"Blame It on the Rain" Milli Vanilli

Our second song with "rain" in the title and also our second song written by Diane Warren, Milli Vanilli's seminal 1989 album *Girl You Know It's True* was, along with Bobby Brown's *My Prerogative*, the first album I got on cassette.* I spent Christmas morning in 1989 rocking out to these cassettes in my new yellow Sony Walkman, smiling and chubby. It is this Christmas morning that I so fondly remember when I'm doing something

---

* Really, the whole *Girl You Know It's True* album is remarkable for its breadth and dexterity, but this song gets the nod in no small part because it inspired the Gulf War–era local radio station parody song "Blame It on Hussein." Man, Saddam Hussein. What a dick.

very adult, like getting my taxes done or buying alcohol or buying alcohol for underage kids.

I am not ashamed to say that I was and still am a huge Milli Vanilli fan. Vacuous pop music that essentially defrauded the entire world? Sure. But do you turn this song off when it comes on your car radio? I rest my case.

When I learned that Milli Vanilli was actually a collection of middle-aged studio musicians and not the chiseled caramel and mocha specimens that I watched dance awkwardly on MTV, I felt a number of emotions. First, there was betrayal. Then sadness. Then guilt. Then not a small amount of hunger. All in, like, twenty seconds. But what I took away most from the Milli Vanilli experience was confusion. At the height of the fiasco, I turned to my mother and forlornly asked, "Mom, why can't they just get the guys who sang on the last album to sing on another album?" She said, "I don't know, Jason. That's just not the way the world works."

And so it was Rob Pilatus and the other, darker one who taught me arguably the most important life lesson of all: fuck you. You may like a song or a band or a friend or a girl or a football team, but in the end, fuck you. Things are not always what they seem to be. Things that are good now will not always be good. And nothing motivates people like personal gain, whether it be in the form of money, power, or fame. When you realize this, you have taken a major step in the transition from adolescence to adulthood.

I am thankful to Rob and the darker one for teaching me this lesson. I am not angry either with them or with the whole situation. I will continue to turn this song up when it comes on my car radio and if I feel any residual anger, I will blame it, of course, on the rain.

(This previous passage is dedicated to the memory of Rob Pilatus, 1965–98. *Atque in perpetuum, frater, ave atque vale.*)

"Over the Hills and Far Away" Led Zeppelin

The first Led Zeppelin songs I heard were what you might expect: "Black Dog," "Stairway to Heaven," "Whole Lotta Love"— those staples of classic rock radio that I heard pour out of roofers' boomboxes as they did work above my head when I walked through the neighborhood on your average summer day. As I began to develop hair on my genitals (around sixth grade—and with the suddenness of a tsunami, if you're keeping score at home), I found myself drawn to the power chords and thunder riffs of Zeppelin, a rite of passage and a badge of manhood for boys my age. But it was this song, with its lovely acoustic intro, that struck me most of all.

This, more than any other, is the song that made me want to start playing guitar. The aforementioned acoustic intro, with its hammer-ons and pull-offs, enchanted me. I could practically see Jimmy Page, taking a break from all his devil worshipping and heroin taking, sitting in a wicker chair in some English farmhouse, playing around and coming up with this introduction. Robert Plant, who would be in the kitchen simultaneously

making some tea and getting fellated, would hear Jimmy playing the intro and walk into the room wearing a pair of jeans
that not only left nothing to the imagination but also looked
like they were suffocating his poor, giant penis. And he'd start
casually singing, "Hey lady . . ." And then: R-O-C-K.

And because I wanted to be Jimmy Page, to sit around with
stoned groupies who adored me and to wear my shirts almost
completely unbuttoned and to say amazingly deep things while
I was high, like "There is love, and there is nothing; it is our
greatest responsibility to make the correct choice," I needed to
learn how to play this song. I needed a guitar. And in eighth
grade on Christmas morning, I got one.

This story is supposed to end with me reaching rock star status—a life filled with gold records, smarmy hangers-on, small
mountains of cocaine, and multiple sexual partners—all from
the humble beginning of lying in bed, listening to the mastery
of Jimmy Page, and masturbating (did I mention this earlier?).
Instead the story of my musical career is one filled with heartbreak, failure, and financial distress. Save for a blow job in the
woods of Vermont after a show at Middlebury College with my
college band (the undeniably untalented Royce), my music career has been one disaster after another. Whether it was repeatedly being told that I "just wasn't that good" or "would never be
more than a below-average rhythm guitarist" or "will be going
to jail if I don't let go of those [genitals] right now", or spending 90 percent of my income between the ages of thirteen and
twenty-two on the latest, greatest, and most expensive guitar
thingy, I now know one thing for certain: the guitar has not
been kind to me. Had I known that Jimmy's sweet intro would

lead me down a path of lowered self-esteem and financial near-ruin, I would have tried a little harder to grow a dragon penis like that of Robert Plant's; I probably had a better chance at becoming well hung than I had of becoming a guitar god.

"Loose Lucy" Grateful Dead

My first concert was a Color Me Badd–Paula Abdul double bill; a better introduction to the power and majesty of live music, I can think of none. My second concert, two years later, was the Grateful Dead.

I was a bona fide Deadhead by the age of twelve. Well, maybe not bona fide—I didn't use drugs or preach love and hippie power—but I was obsessed with the Dead. There was a time when both Jimmy the Muppet and I could name all twenty-eight Dead albums released to that point. Among those albums, *From the Mars Hotel* was high on my list of favorites. "Loose Lucy" in particular stood out on that album for me, probably because of its racy implications. Even at the age of twelve, I knew that *loose* meant "whorish," so that was certainly exciting. But there was also the theory that "Loose Lucy" was not a woman at all but similar to the Lucy in the sky with those diamonds that the Beatles had sung about, a possibility I found equally enticing. Advice to bands: if you're looking to tap into the male preteen/early teen demographic, secretly suggest that your song is about sluts and drugs. Works every time.

Luckily for me, the Dead played "Loose Lucy" when I saw

them in concert at the old Philadelphia Spectrum. But it was not what happened during the concert that so influenced my adolescence (even though watching an overweight, zonked-out Jerry Garcia hunched over his guitar for two and a half hours was pretty awesome), but rather what happened before the concert, outside in the parking lot of the Spectrum. It was there that for the first time, in person, I saw a boob.

It was only a quick glimpse, but one never forgets their first booby. It came courtesy of a fairly chestily blessed but otherwise waifish Deadhead, a blonde who couldn't have been more than twenty years old. She was not flashing the crowd, flaunting her breasts for all to see. If this had been the case, I would have felt uncomfortable (in addition to feeling hard, of course). Instead she was merely walking around the parking lot, her one finger in the air, looking for that one magic ticket to get her into the show. I didn't notice her until she was upon my friends and I, who were desperately trying to score nitrous.* As she walked by me, coming toward me on my right, I turned to look at her. It was her right hand that was in the air, creating a spectacular view through the armpit of her loose-fitting hippie dress, and there it was—a small, supple, pale white booby, no bigger than a fist. It dangled on her chest, unencumbered by a bra. I was transfixed. In that instant, it was just me and that booby. No one else—not my friends, not other concertgoers, not even the owner of the booby herself—noticed it gloriously perched above her slender

---

* I mean, how could a drug that comes in a balloon possibly be harmful for a twelve-year-old?

lil' 'shroom and veggie burrito–filled stomach. Just the booby and I, sharing a secret moment, creating a special memory, one that I recall each time I hear that opening riff of Jerry's guitar and that first line, "Loose Lucy is my delight."

A better introduction to the power and majesty of breasts, I can think of none.

Chapter Nine

My Bird: Inadequacy and Redemption

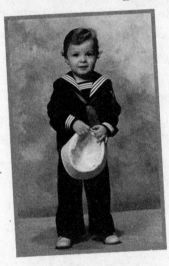

Apparently, the cop and construction worker costumes were in the cleaners.

I have always been concerned with the diminutive size of my penis. I blame this on two things: Carlos Flores and the chip.

Carlos Flores was the only Hispanic kid in my first-grade

class of ninety or so kids.* Actually, he was the only minority in the whole class; there were eighty-nine kids of Irish, Polish, Lithuanian, or Italian descent (or some combination thereof) and then ol' Carlos Fucking Flores. Shockingly, he did not return to Our Lady of Mount Carmel for second grade, but in his short time at OLMC, Carlos Flores changed my life.

I was peeing next to Carlos at a urinal when he turned and looked at me peeing and said, "What are you doing?" I don't remember my exact response but I'm guessing it was "Um, taking a pee?" followed by complete and horrified silence at having another kid talk to me while we were peeing. Regardless of my response, Carlos, who probably has a successful career in journalism now, followed up his first bold question with a second equally daring question: "Why are you holding it like *that*?"

The "it," of course, was my penis—or as we called it in my family, my bird. I don't know why my family gave such an innocuous name to something that would cause me such a great amount of mental and emotional distress—not to mention cost me over $480—later in life, but the etymology of *bird* is a discussion for another day. Carlos was waiting for an answer. I looked down at my penis, looking especially thimble-like in my soft, delicate, six-year-old hands. I looked at Carlos, confused.

"Why are you holding it like this," he said while emulating my grip on my penis, "when you should do it like this," and gripped his penis the "proper" way.

---

* I do not know what nationality Carlos was for certain. My dad met his dad at a parent-teacher conference and described him as being from "one of those Puerto Rico–type countries," so I guess we'll just go with that.

In this instant, I learned two important life lessons:

1. **I am a pincher.** Have you ever seen one of those animal shows on the Discovery Channel that show footage of mother lions carrying their cubs in their mouths? It looks very painful for the baby lion, what with his mother biting him around the nape of the neck, roughly picking him up, and then carrying him for a little while. But it's not.* I know this because this is how I grabbed—and still grab—my penis when I urinate. I hold it by taking the skin from the side of my penis between my thumb and forefinger, pinching that skin, lifting the penis and letting it dangle below my fingers while urinating, just like a lion cub who cries out as his mother drags him by her teeth around the plains of the Serengeti. I thought this was the only way to hold a bird while one is peeing, but Carlos demonstrated to me that the "real" way to hold one was to cradle it in one's hand, and not like the mother lion holding her weary cub in her teeth with her clenched jaw but (to continue with our wildlife kingdom analogies) more like a retarded boy handling a sleeping hamster— lovingly, and with a delicateness that is inspired by a complicated mix of fear, confusion, and awe. "See? Not like your way, but like my way," he said, wagging his penis, which was no longer urinating, in his hand in

---

* Note: I have absolutely no scientific or even fictional research to back this up.

front of the urinal next to mine. Which brings us to the second lesson I learned:

2. **Carlos Flores had a penis the size of a table leg.** It was giant, gargantuan. I did not then nor do not now have the words to describe it. It looked less like a penis and more like a weapon, like it had a purpose greater than peeing, like hitting Wiffle balls or knocking holes in Sheetrock. It needed a name, not a cute one like Mr. Willy or Captain Pee-Pee, but something like Max Strong America or James Bond Powerful Justice or God's Tougher Friend Steve. It was larger than the Little Hug juices we drank at lunch, it was larger than the erasers we used on the chalkboard during class, it was larger than the remote control I used to turn on the TV after school. For weeks after this incident—hell, years even—I thought about whether what Carlos had was even a penis at all or perhaps another living thing growing out of his groin. Looking at it, I wouldn't have been surprised if it took out a cigarette, lit it, and then asked me what I thought about that "anarcho-syndicalist bastard" Noam Chomsky before telling me I really needed to invest in a good pair of slacks. It was a force. It was respect, genitalized.

After being treated to Carlos's gorilla-bird, I again examined my own bird, which looked even smaller now than it had before I saw his. I had not seen another penis before, so I had nothing to compare mine to. But the differences were clear after that encounter at the urinal. Carlos's penis was a highlighter; mine was a pen cap. Carlos's was a lightbulb; mine was a light switch.

Carlos's was the thermos that clanged around all day long in my lunch box; mine was the Hershey Kiss that had melted sometime during social studies.

Carlos, God bless his Puerto Rican–type heart, made no mention of my penile inadequacy. He zipped up, flushed, and promptly walked out of the bathroom and back to class. But he didn't need to say anything else. For the first time, I realized that my dick was tiny. If Carlos's penis was what other guys' birds looked like, I was in for a lifetime of emotional pain and humiliation. Mind you, this was before I knew that penises were for sex, and yet I *still* was horribly dismayed by the inadequate size of mine, based on my preternatural understanding that in all things, bigger was better. What I had dangling between (or rather, sticking out above) my legs was not up to par. From this point forward, my life would be nothing more than a litany of excuses and apologies on account of my lil' bird, whether they be directed to the women I'd be unable to please, or those frat brothers who paid me fourteen dollars to see it in 2006.[*]

I may not remember my first day of class, the days either of my siblings were born, or even my first kiss. But I will always remember seeing Carlos's ginormous hog at the urinal next to mine in first grade. The doubts that his Powerade bottle–penis instilled in me would remain with me for years, and would be buttressed when my family made the decision to get "the chip," thus heightening my hysteria and all but confirming my greatest fear.[**]

---

[*] Again, sorry about that, Mike, Matt, and Cam.
[**] Greatest non-werewolf-related fear, that is.

* * *

Whether the chip was an actual chip or a code or a cut wire, I'm not sure. Regardless, it was a contrivance that allowed a household to steal cable. How it worked was that one of your uncle's friends, usually a shady alcoholic quite like your uncle, came into your house and finagled with your cable box. After hitting on the woman of the house and drinking five beers in twenty minutes, he'd take his $120 fee and it was all done. That household now had unlimited access to all the premium cable channels, like HBO, Showtime, and Cinemax. Not only that, but the chip also gave free access to pay-per-view events like boxing and wrestling and such. And, most important, the chip meant that I now had access to not one, not two, but *three* porno channels: the Playboy Channel (channel 35), Adam & Eve (channel 77), and the Spice Channel (channel 78).

In sixth grade, my family got the chip, one of the first in the neighborhood to do so.* At that age, I felt about porn the same

---

* Soon, almost everyone in the neighborhood had the chip, a development that would give birth to one of the greatest childhood games of my or any era: remote controlling. All the houses in my neighborhood were row homes, stacked against each other, without front or back lawns, and with windows and screen doors that opened directly into their homes. Often, curtains, blinds, and storm doors were left open, exposing an intimate view to passersby of the home's living room—a couch here, some kids laying on the floor over there, a dad sitting in his chair there, and in the middle of it all, a television.

    My friends and I would take the remote controls from our houses and roam the streets of the neighborhood looking for the perfect home to sabotage—one that had a clear view to the TV and living room, with a family sitting around watching the local news or *Wheel of Fortune* or something. Banking on the fact that this home probably had the chip, we'd point our remote controls at their TV and change the channel to one of the porno channels. If the family didn't have the chip, the channel would turn way I felt about crack: it was out there, it was dangerous, and it would ultimately ruin you. Blame this on my Irish Catholic upbringing and schooling, but pornography scared the hell out of me, especially when I knew I had unlimited access to it. Evil was right there, in my own home, and its presence alone nearly drove me to confession. I wanted no part of pornography.

That is until, you know, I actually started watching it.

One day after school, with my sister with a babysitter, my brother who knows where*, and my mother at work, curiosity got the best of me and I turned to channel 78, the Spice Channel, just to take a peek.

Less than two seconds after putting it on, I changed the channel away from the Spice Channel. That brief glimpse of porn was a standard girl-on-girl scene, one that I've seen about a million times since (and about thirty to forty times today). But this first exposure was shocking. One thing I later learned about the Spice Channel in comparison to the Playboy Channel (which didn't show penetration) and the Adam & Eve channel (which didn't show "pop shots"—the man ejaculating on the woman's stomach, back, chest, face, eyes, or hair) is that the Spice Channel didn't pull any punches. It was far and away the most

---

to static. If they did, they'd miss the answer to Final Jeopardy because some twenty-one-year-old with fake tits was now on the TV screen guzzling cum with a big smile on her face. Watching the confusion that unfolded after successfully changing the channel—everyone jumping up from their seats, running to change the channel, completely befuddled as to what happened, screaming and yelling and cursing—is one of my most treasured memories. If there is a heaven, and if I get in after I die, I'll spend 90 percent of my time going remote controlling with my childhood friends.

* Probably at the hoagie factory. God, he was so fat as a kid.

X-rated of the three channels. When I turned to channel 78, I was treated to a giant close-up of a vagina, being less than lovingly caressed by another woman. I still consider vaginas one of the most terrifying things on the planet,* so this extreme close-up of a region that I barely knew existed was not an ideal introduction to the female sex. Then and there, I made a promise that I would never put on the porno channel again.

And for a few days, I didn't. But the next time I had the whole house to myself, I tuned in again. On that afternoon, I learned two more important life lessons:

1. **This whole "free porn" thing was going to work out just fine.** Once I got over my initial jitters, I sat there Indian-style on the floor, flipping between channels 35, 77, and 78, watching different scenes and different scenarios, taking it all in, learning, growing, living, and nearly ripping my poor penis off (after the second round, it became unclear whether I was masturbating or seizing). I'm surprised that detectives from the Special Victims Unit didn't show up at my door and arrest me for penile endangerment. I actually don't even like talking about this, since I still feel a tremendous amount of guilt for my actions on that afternoon. It got a little out of control.

2. **What I suspected before was now official: I had the smallest bird in the world.** While I never forgot the lesson I had learned the day Carlos Flores showed me his

---

* Right up there with sharks, the previously mentioned werewolves, and pretty much everyone on BET.

forearm-esque penis, I had finally been able to push it to the back of my mind. My small bird would forever be my cross to bear, but it was also still my secret—Carlos had left school and taken the events of that day with him, and since then I hadn't been in a situation where someone saw my bird. In time, I thought about my little penis less and less.

But porn changed all that. The guys in the pornos that I watched that afternoon had not penises, but *PENISES*. Like Carlos, their birds seemed to be not mere appendages, but rather freestanding entities that could make positive contributions to society under the right circumstances, as carpenters, karate instructors, or politicians.

And the women in the pornos were obviously enjoying these penises. What I found menacing, they thought was just the tops. Now that I was old enough to realize that my bird would eventually be counted on to make a woman happy (or at least not completely bored and/or shameful), the notion that women wanted giant dicks depressed the hell out of me. How would I ever be able to please a woman with this half-pinkie I had for a bird? What woman would be able to find enjoyment from something that she needed to find with a flashlight and a pair of eyebrow tweezers? Not only that, would I even be able to have sex at all? The mechanics of sex confused me. How would I, with what I had, even be able to get the proper amount of penetration necessary to establish the very basics of sex? From what I learned from the porno channels, in my case it would be like sticking a Jolly Rancher into a bowl of oatmeal.

These questions would haunt me, keep me awake at night, make me doubt my very manhood. Until my thief friend helped me answer them.

Stealing was what Ronnie White did best. It seemed like each kid in my eighth-grade class had a personality trait or hobby that defined him or her—Timmy Cooper the Gay, Cheryl Baker the Girl with Giant Boobs, Chris Turner the Kid That Fell off Batting Cages, Janine Harris the Black Girl—and Ronnie was definitely the Thief. Ronnie looked like a marine, with his crew cut, his thin, wiry frame, and his intense gaze, but he was a very affable guy whose ability to laugh at himself made him fun to be around. And of course, there was the stealing.

Ronnie stole *everything*. He was just as likely to rob Tower Records of CDs and movies as he was to steal plastic hangers and cough medicine from CVS. There was really no limit to what he'd pinch. On the same Saturday, he'd walk out of Foot Locker wearing a new pair of shorts, steal a plant from Home Depot, and swipe a ream of construction paper from Staples. But he truly never stole for utility. Ronnie stole for the fun of it and to get a laugh out of us, his friends. The more random the item he stole, the more we laughed when he told us about it.

Kmart was a favorite victim of Ronnie's, filled as it was with such a variety of items. Stereos, pizza, shampoo, tank tops—all of it could be found at the Kmart at Third and Oregon, smack in the middle of the area where we spent most of our time. It was in the parking lot of the Kmart on a Sunday afternoon in fall that Ronnie pulled out his latest booty: a royal blue box of

Trojan condoms. None of us had seen condoms before, but we knew how important they were. To have sex, you needed to wear a condom.* In essence, if you had a condom, you were halfway to sex (more or less). Ronnie ripped open the box and gave each of us present—me, and my friends Ernie and Hutton—three condoms each. In that moment, we became Men.

The four of us would not need to use a condom for many years,** but the very fact that we owned them, that we had them at our disposal should the need arise, instantly made us more confident and more adult. I was not thinking of the long-term implications of condom ownership, but rather focusing on the immediate future. The only way to resolve the question that had haunted me for years—was my bird big enough?—was to try on one of these condoms. If the condom fit, my penis and I would be fine. If not, there would be a problem, one that would be resolved with either an entrance into the priesthood or a bottle of whiskey, a butter knife, and a Ken doll to use as a model. This was a matter that needed to be addressed right now.

And so I thanked Ronnie, bid my friends good-bye, and headed for that familiar place where I spent the majority of my adolescent sex life—the cold tile floor of the bathroom. I disrobed into what would become my preferred level of nudity for

---

* I'm not sure if this mandate was a product of Irish Catholic education, which traditionally doesn't favor any sort of birth control, or my Uncle Tommy, who at every Thanksgiving since I was old enough to hear would get drunk and tell me, "Jason, for Chrissake, just wear a condom. Trust me."

** And I don't think ever for Hutton—not because he didn't have sex, but because he is sterile and he also doesn't believe in STDs.

sex for many years—no pants or underwear, but with a shirt and socks on.*

I studied the condom in the wrapper and was surprised at how easy it was to open it.** Once I removed it from the wrapper, I was also surprised at how terrible it smelled—in the spectrum of nasty smells, latex covered in spermicide is right up there with "garbage fire" and "testicles after eight hours working the grill at Chili's." The whole experience left me feeling quite unaroused, but as I was thirteen years old, a quick flashback to that day in gym class when in the process of falling and spraining her ankle Cheryl Baker's boob nearly fell out fixed me right up and I was bonerized in no time. Now it was time for the reckoning.

As I would do four more times in my life, I put the condom on my penis. I didn't have the instructions but figured it out rather quickly because as a young child I used to store my socks away by rolling them up like doughnuts and putting them in the dresser, so that when I put them on all I had to do was place them on the my feet and roll them up. The condom worked the same way. There, half naked and lying on the bathroom floor, I placed the condom on top of my bird, which seemed frightened by the whole experience and looking for a way to escape, and slowly started rolling the condom down. And—

It fit.

I rolled it down until I couldn't anymore, but the condom,

---

* I like to leave some clothes on in case I get cold.

** I always thought they'd be tough to open, like how you'd see in movies or TV shows, so learning that they were easy to open was quite a relief and allowed me to fret about other sex-related issues, namely, "Where does my bird go again?"

which I feared would hang loosely on my penis like a toga, gripped my bird snugly. I tugged on it a bit to see if it would slide off, but it did not budge. I stood up, fearing the movement of my body might cause it to fall off, but it did not budge. Erect but getting softer, I shook my hips and swung my condom-covered penis back and forth, but it did not budge. That condom was not going anywhere. Because it fit.

After years of mental torment and hundreds of sleepless nights, my concerns about the size of my penis were erased in one afternoon. That the condom fit meant that my bird met the minimum standard of penis size among American men. Fathers, lock up your daughters.

Chapter Ten

Guns. Fucking Guns.

Guns are cool. This is one of the basic premises we operated under as kids, right up there with *Yes, I'll have some more Pepsi* and *Nintendo is better than homework*. Now I'm a bleeding-heart liberal and the very mention of guns sends me screaming into the nearest bathroom, where I will shit and cry until someone assures me that no, there are no guns around. But when I was a mere child, I loved me some guns.

I don't think I really need to explain the appeal of the gun, but we have some time to kill here, so I might as well give it a shot.* Most of the people I wanted to be as a kid—cowboys, GI Joe, James Bond, innumerable video game characters—used

---

* Get it? "Shot"? Maybe I shouldn't have written so much of this after three in the morning.

guns and did so with extreme prejudice. This was back when the desire to inflict death and destruction were normal impulses for a child and wouldn't warrant an intervention or trip to the child psychologist. To wit: I was a cowboy for at least three of my first seven Halloweens, using my pump action (cap) shotgun to mow down the lesser Cookie Monsters, She-Ras, and even Bat-men (I wasn't buying the whole "bulletproof face cream" thing; if I shoot Batman in the face, he's going down). Toy guns were a go-to gift, one that would never fail to disappoint. I don't think a single birthday or Christmas passed between 1979 and 1993 that I didn't get something that I could use to fake-kill something else.

(And don't even get me started on water guns. Sure, maybe they were a bit lame, what with water rather than bullets raining terror upon enemies, but we didn't *have* any bullets. Water guns at least let us know that we were hitting our adversaries, and the Super Soakers' streams of water proved to us that we were obliterating our enemies. When Super Soakers were released in 1991, I slept with mine every night until college. There were three main technological advances of my youth that changed me forever when they debuted: Sega Genesis, Upper Deck base-ball cards, and the Super Soaker. I don't think, in terms of inno-vation, America has seen anything before or since like the three years in which these were released.)

What made guns even more appealing was that they were so *forbidden*. Later in life, when I met and made friends with people who never asked for a glass of *wudder* and didn't respond to the question "Did you eat?" by saying "Nah, jew?" I learned that some people grew up around guns. That is, not only were guns displayed in their homes, not only were they accessible, but these people, as children, were actually taught to shoot guns (!). I cannot fathom what would have happened if this were the case in my home. I'm pretty sure that I would no longer have a brother and my little sister would have only one arm or would otherwise have been chased out of the house to join a troupe of Gypsies, frightened off by my shotgun blasts.

Fortunately for my brother and sister, guns were not accessible in our house. But they were present. My dad had guns and I knew this, but I was only vaguely aware of them. Prior to the divorce, my dad had a box in his and my mom's bedroom closet,

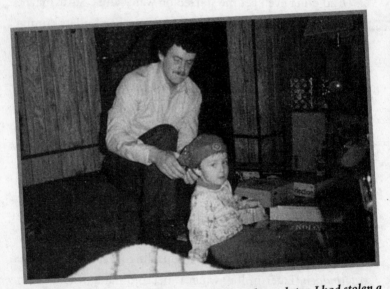

My dad preparing me for gang warfare. Four hours later, I had stolen a car stereo and shivved three Dominicans.

a cross between an oversized jewelry box and a safe. In it, I assumed, were his guns. I was never explicitly told this but was repeatedly warned to stay the hell away from the box. The most dangerous thing that my six-year-old brain could conjure being in the box was guns. In retrospect, it could have been anything from guns to drugs to porn. Now I have a similar box in my own bedroom closet but there are no guns in there. Lots of lots of movies of black people fucking each other at frat parties, but no guns.

As I got older (or as he got crazier), my dad was less concerned with concealing his weapons from my siblings and me. After my parents' divorce was settled, just after my family and I moved back into our house after living with my grandmother for over two years, my dad moved out and around a lot, going from one seedy neighborhood to another. He must have changed apartments four times in three years, but there was one thing he always had wherever he lived: his elephant gun.

The elephant gun was a giant, single-shot rifle that stood as tall as I did, weighed as much as my little sister, and used bullets the size of a grown man's middle finger. My dad said that it was used to hunt elephants, so my brother and I called it (naturally) the elephant gun. This was always kept behind whatever couch my dad had in whatever living room he was living in. For some reason (possibly marijuana-induced), my dad allowed my brother and me to play with the elephant gun. But don't go saying that my dad was an irresponsible parent; he made sure to unload the gun before every visit. Except that day when I spent most of one lazy afternoon aiming the gun at my brother, Dennis, who was then six, before my dad took it from me, because, I can only assume, I was being obnoxious. When he did so, he realized that there was a bullet in the chamber. Oops. This remains one of the only times I've ever seen my dad rattled. His face turned pale and after a moment of reflection, once he recognized what a mistake he had made, he asked us not to tell our mother. We obliged. Looking back, if I had told my mom about this, at this delicate time in their divorce, I may have never seen my dad again.* Instead, now every time I get drunk, sleepwalk, and piss in my dad's hallway, I only have to say, "Remember when I almost killed Dennis because you didn't unload your gun?" and I get a free pass.**

My dad finally settled into a place on Beulah Street. There, behind a hutch that was designed to hold china but instead housed bottles of Smirnoff and Courvoisier, stood some sort of samurai axe. Also tall, though not as big as the elephant gun (the axe was about the size of my brother), it was a double-sided axe with a bladelike spear on top. I have no idea how my dad got this or why he had it, but my brother and I were allowed to play with this, supervised of course, as well. But in my dad's defense, I seem to remember the blades looking pretty dull, so I'm sure if would have done only minimal damage to my brother's neck/shoulders/arms/balls if I struck him with it.

---

* This is me being dramatic, but it would not have been very good for my dad had my mom learned about the loaded gun incident.

** This is a lie. If I pissed in my dad's house, he would make me eat the piss-covered carpet and would then take me outside and run me over with his truck. So the more fitting example would be something like, "Every time I use the last of the milk and my dad gets pissed at me . . ."

The ever-present danger and the fact that my dad had guns only made me want them more. I carried a cap gun on me constantly until about age ten, partially to feel cool, but partially because I believed it really protected me. When I was old enough, I graduated from toy guns to "real" weapons. In seventh grade, my friends and I started carrying around "blackjacks." These were made by breaking off one of the long, thin pieces of wood under the chairs of our school desks. We'd take this piece, which looked like a shorter, thicker wooden ruler, and pile pennies along the length of it, four pennies high in a row of seven. Then, using black hockey tape, we'd tape the pennies down to the piece of wood, first lengthwise to secure them, then by wrapping the tape around the wood. The end product was a mobile but effective weapon that could easily be hidden down one's pants or in one's waistband. Theoretically, we carried the blackjacks in case we got jumped. We believed that this was a constant threat in the neighborhood—that a group of kids from another corner would grab you and fuck you up.* If you were going to get jumped, there was very little you could do to avoid it. You had two options: either name-drop like a mother fucker, saying your brother/cousin/sister's boyfriend was [insert badass dude here] or call out one of the guys in the group about to

---

* There was precedent for this: Eclipse was the first guy any of us knew who got jumped. He was returning a video to West Coast Video when a group of kids from Avenue and Morris grabbed him, beat him up, and stole his video. The two things that most stand out in my mind about this was the name of the video (the Tom Hanks classic tearjerker *Turner & Hooch*) and how much West Coast Video charged Eclipse's mom for the lost video ($92).

jump you and offer to fight him one-on-one. However, rarely was there so much thinking involved and you just got beat the fuck up. So essentially the blackjack was useless, as it did almost nothing to combat getting jumped. Sure, you might be able to brandish it, but when a half dozen or a dozen kids are descending on you, there isn't much you can do, blackjack or not. But hey, at least the blackjacks made us feel cool.

A pair of brass knuckles was my next step up from the blackjack. I don't know how I came across a pair—I'm sure it must have had something to do with someone's older brother who got them from someone else but who was now selling them for money for beer/weed/pills. I used them, of all places, on my paper route, which was two blocks away from my street and one block away from my church. I guess I wanted to be prepared in case any thugs came out of the ten o'clock mass looking to start some shit.

After reading what I've written so far, I need to interject here for a moment and clear something up. While I may sound like a little "street tough," walking my paper route with my brass knuckles close by in case any shit went down, nothing could be further from the truth. In reality, I was a chubby twelve-year-old who had only kissed one girl and spent most of his disposal income on comic books and most of his time exploring the new and wonderful world of masturbation, slathering himself up with moisturizer and going to town. It was a charmed life, really. But perhaps that is why my friends and I were so into weapons. The lure of the weapon, the desire to possess the weapon, and the longing for others to know that you possessed the weapon was a universal truth in my youth. Guns and our other weapons represented a power that was otherwise out of our collective grasp as stupid kids.

But we were just that. Stupid fucking kids.

I had a kind of love/hate relationship with my buddies Phil and Vic. On the one hand, they were two of my closest friends. We did almost everything together, although admittedly "almost everything" consisted mostly of sitting around the Park, hanging out, and waiting for some friends to get in a fight over a pickup basketball game. Then there was that week when we were catching and blowing up mice with my leftover firecrackers. That was pretty cool.

But they were unconscionable ballbusters. Phil was a great basketball player and never hesitated to tell you about it. Though he had a good sense of humor, he was a tough and competitive kid and could be abrasive, to put it mildly. As a twelve-year-old, Vic weighed almost two hundred pounds and had fists the size of Easter hams. He was considered a gentle giant with an encyclopedic knowledge of classic rock, but at the same time he seemed like he could go off at any moment. And god *damn* he was a big dude. Then there was me. I didn't play any sports (didn't play any sports well, at least), was chubby but not intimidating, and spent my time talking to the girls, desperately trying to make them laugh, and by extension, desperately trying to get them to let me touch them under their bras. The former I was good at; the latter, well, not so much.*

Therefore, as the "weakest" member of the three of us, I was often the victim of Phil's and Vic's bullying tendencies. It seemed like every time it snowed, I was the one who got white-washed (held down and packed with snow) first and most maliciously. We used to pillow-box, wrapping pillows around our fists in place of boxing gloves, but it seemed like the pillows slipped off Phil's and Vic's hands more when they were fighting me than when they were fighting others, leaving me bruised up and sometimes with a fat lip.

[Note to reader: The following paragraph should be read in the style of Ray Liotta, reprising his role as narrator and protagonist Henry Hill in *Goodfellas*.]

Yet I didn't mind. I was still in the crew. There was me, Phil, Vic, Floody, Jimmy the Muppet, Eclipse, and Screech. Then there were guys like Ernie Bubble, Hutt, Brown Eye, Eddie C., Chad, Kruzer, Doc, Renzi, Robbie C, Patty K., Adam, Coast to Coast Steve Trusko, Big J., Beaver, Large, and the Wigs. We may have disagreed with each other and had the occasional fight, but we were a family.

[Here ends the Ray Liotta/Henry Hill voice.]

An occasional whitewash wasn't a sign of disrespect and didn't mean I wasn't part of this extended family. We busted the balls of our friends; we *picked on* people outside our circle. Like Danny Kramer, whom we covered so thoroughly with ketchup and creamer from Burger King that he started crying. So we locked him in the bathroom of the local pool hall for an

---

* I've gotten better though, thanks mostly to tequila.

afternoon. And there was Shitty Brian, so named because he got the Shit Nose. On his way home from karate, a group of my friends grabbed him, held him down, and the nastiest of the bunch put their bare asses on his face, thus proving once and for all that karate is for pussies—he wasn't karate chopping any blocks of wood when he had ass on his face. Snow in your ears was not a big deal. Shit on your face was. This was an important distinction.

I dealt with Phil and Vic being dicks every once in a while because we were boys. I knew that I wasn't being disrespected, it wasn't something that was constant, and there was no real physical pain, so I didn't think much of it. Or maybe I'm just rationalizing their abuse because I was (and still am) a total pussy. That could be true, but then there's also this: fuck you.

A big part of the friendship that Vic and I shared was our love for music. He had an older brother, and while the rest of us were listening to MC Hammer and Poison, Vic's brother was feeding him a steady diet of the Beatles, Led Zeppelin, and the Grateful Dead. It was at Vic's family's house up the mountains* that I was first introduced to the *other* music of the Beatles. I had heard "Ticket to Ride" and "I Want to Hold Your Hand" before while my mom cleaned the house. But when Vic gave me *Sgt. Pepper's Lonely Hearts Club Band* to listen to in my brand-new portable CD player, I, like about two hundred million other people before me, had an awakening. From then on, Vic became my musical mentor, turning me on to all sorts

---

* Going "up the mountains" meant a trip to the Poconos, just as going "down the shore" meant a vacation in North Wildwood, NJ.

of different stuff that wasn't made by any former members of New Edition.

And Phil—well, girls liked Phil.

That Phil went to tennis camp was an anomaly. Tennis was not a sport played in the neighborhood. The only acceptable sports were basketball, football, baseball, and hockey. They could be played in different incarnations (that is, flag football, Wiffle ball, etc.), but these were the four sports. There was a brief flirtation with soccer when the World Cup came to the United States in 1994, but we're talking very brief—it ended when the volleyball we were using as a soccer ball was lost.

Phil might have been on to something though, because what going to tennis camp meant was exposure to new girls. Frankly, we were all sick of the girls from the neighborhood.* The Second Street girls were divided into two groups, the Pretty Girls and the ASP. The Pretty Girls were, as the name implies, attractive. They were the first girls to start wearing makeup and high heels and bras and, I don't know, whatever girls wear when they're growing up and first learning how to manipulate their sexuality. The Pretty Girls were out of our league, preferring instead to date older guys (you know, like high school guys). Naturally, we resented them. ASP stood for "Ankle Sock Posse," referring to the athletic short socks that the girls in this group wore to

---

* Not me, though. Really, any and all girls were okay with me. As much as I liked masturbating on the bathroom floor, I aspired to bigger and better and warmer things.

play basketball. The girls of the ASP preferred mesh shorts and ponytails to heels and makeup and had seemingly zero interest in exploring their sexuality.* But still, they were cool girls who could handle it when one of us walked over to them holding a piece of his scrotum in his hand from under his mesh shorts and asked, "Does anyone want a piece of Juicy Fruit? I chewed it up a bit, but it's still good." But romantically speaking, we lusted after the Pretty Girls, whom we couldn't have; we hung out with the ASP, whom we didn't want.**

At tennis camp, Phil had a pipeline into new girls, who my friends and I automatically assumed were prettier than our girls and also more liable to put out. After the first summer when he returned from the camp, he regaled us with stories of the girls there, of discreet hand jobs (or at least knob rubs) in the woods and of campfire make-out sessions. But Phil being Phil, we didn't know if this was true or if it was only his braggadocio talking. We treated his stories with the proper skepticism, asking for proof, which he not so surprisingly could not provide.

After his second summer at tennis camp, Phil returned with more of the same stories, but this time he came back with

---

*The girls of the ASP would eventually grow up to be beautiful women. Perhaps I'm just bitter because while I was at my sexual peak at the ripe old age of twelve, they were more interested in boxing out and foul shots than they were in getting felt up by me.

**The boys were also divided, into the Pretty Boys and the Roughnecks. The Pretty Boys were like their female counterparts; they wore Drakkar, put gel in their hair, and wore gold chains. Basically anybody who wasn't a Pretty Boy was considered a Roughneck, a wide group that encompassed everything from jocks to aspiring drunkards/stoners to normal guys. I was a Roughneck.

something else—a telephone number. It belonged to a girl named Adriana (such an exotic name!) whom he had met and made out with at camp. He told us first that she was hot and had large boobies, but also that her dad was a judge. (A judge! She must be rich! And rich girls put out! Probably!) The collective awe of the crowd was nearly audible.

Vic and I were eager to tap into this new resource. The girls of the neighborhood knew us and wanted nothing to do with us, but this, this was opportunity knocking. Perhaps I could meet a nice rich girl, get a bunch of hand jobs, get married, and then buy a house with a nice big pool. That would be nice. So it was Vic and I who were chosen to accompany Phil on a group date to the movies with Adriana and her girlfriends.* *Chosen* might not be the right word, since from the moment he brought up the possibility of a group date, Vic and I badgered him about going. The plan was that Phil, Vic, and I would meet Adriana and her friends at the movies. Phil would pair off with Adriana while Vic and I would be left to go after her friends. After the movie, we'd all go get a slice of pizza. If it all worked out, we'd make out in the parking lot of the pizza place, which would be the most sexually advanced thing I'd ever done to that point by tenfold.

Prior to the date, Vic got ready by listening to Steely Dan.

---

* A year or two earlier, a new cineplex had opened in the neighborhood. This was a modern technological marvel and for a few months after its opening, everyone became serious moviegoers. Prior to this cineplex's opening, we had to travel over the Walt Whitman Bridge to Jersey to find the nearest movie theater. More important, next to the theater opened a rock-'n'-roll-themed restaurant with fifteen-cent wings and twenty different kinds of milkshakes. Then it burned down. I miss that place.

He shaved, which was a privilege and obvious sign of manliness among twelve-year-olds. When he was finished, he got dressed, sat in the leather recliner he and his brother had in their cramped room, and secretly smoked a cigarette out his window.

I did not shave before the date, because I did not have any hair to shave.* I did, however, obsessively brush my teeth, so concerned was I with kissing a girl while having bad breath. When I finished, I sat down on my bed and listened to John Lennon sing "Cry Baby Cry" to help me calm down. This was going to be a good night. I hoped.

Phil, much more accustomed to these types of things than either Vic or I, threw on a splash of cologne (likely Drakkar) when he stepped out of the shower. He put on his nice new Structure shirt, tousled his hair, checked himself in the mirror, and, as a final touch, put his gun in his pants. He was ready to go out.

A few weeks before, Phil had bought a gun. A fake gun, that is. We were too old for cap guns but not nearly old enough for the real thing, so this particular gun was somewhere in the middle. It was a replica gun, like an inoperative model of a gun. It shot neither caps nor bullets—it shot nothing, actually. He bought it because it looked alarmingly like a real gun. Phil had taken to carrying around his "piece," as he called it, everywhere. I couldn't blame him; it was a pretty fucking cool gun, a chrome .38 revolver, nice and new and shiny. But what was different about this gun from other fake guns was not only how real it looked, but how real it *felt*. Phil's gun had some real weight to it, and unless you knew it was a fake, you would never guess it was.

---

* Sweet, sweet youth!

As Phil, Vic, and I walked to the movie theater to the meet the girls, Phil lifted his shirt, showing us the gun in his waistband. Vic and I rolled our eyes, thinking this was Phil trying to be his usual "badass" self, and didn't think anything else about it. There were more important things to worry about tonight.

At the movies we met Adriana, Phil's interest, and, for me and Vic to divide and conquer, Christine and Faith. It was plain to see early on in the evening that neither Vic nor I would be sharing a glorious make-out session with either girl. Just as we had begged/forced Phil to bring us along, it seems that Adriana had begged/forced Christine and Faith to come along with her. Actually, I don't think any of the four of them—Phil, Adriana, Christine, and Faith—spoke to either Vic or me all night. Adriana deferred to Phil, adoringly almost, as he aced the audition before Christine and Faith. Vic and I talked to each other, but rarely. At best we came off as strong silent types; at worst we looked like Phil's bodyguards/semiretarded friends.

After the movie, during which Phil and Adriana made out with each other the entire time flanked by Vic and me on one side and Christine and Faith on the other, we stuck to the original plan and went to get pizza. The pizza place was only a block away, a store in a small strip mall that also contained a Wawa,* a check-cashing place, a video store, and an empty store. There was a large parking lot in front of these stores and opposite the stores on the other side of the parking lot were two busy gas stations. This area was just underneath an exit off Interstate 95, the

* Wawa is like the Philadelphia area's version of 7-Eleven, but much, much cleaner.

main north-south artery on the east coast of the United States, and which runs right through Philadelphia.

Vic and I watched Phil and the girls carry on at the pizza place. We laughed when it seemed appropriate to laugh but mostly kept to ourselves. I was bummed out by the whole situation but had long before given up on the night. I had had high hopes heading into it, but the coldness of Christine and Faith brought them crashing to the ground. I did not consider myself the next Warren Beatty, but a little nonaccidental eye contact would have been nice. So as I still do when I face rejection from women, I shut down. Fuck it, I thought, if they don't want to talk to me, I don't want to talk them. They're probably lesbians anyway. Yeah, lesbos. Eff them.

After we finished the pizza, the guys, chivalrous as we were, got up to pay for the slices and sodas. Vic and I, as we were sitting on the outside seats, got up first, but Phil told us to sit down. "Guys, I got it," he said as he lifted up his shirt to show the girls his gun.

Seeing the girls squirm with fright, Phil quickly added, "Nah—I'm just kidding! It's fake!" He pulled the gun out of his pants and plopped it on the table for them to see. Adriana and Christine were fascinated by the gun and how real it looked, asking various questions that Phil answered coolly and mysteriously ("Where did you get it?" "I got it from a buddy." "How much was it?" "Don't worry about it, but not cheap."). Vic and I rolled our eyes and wished that we were more athletic, or at least good at tennis. Faith was very uncomfortable with the gun. Even though she was told it was a harmless fake, it looked too authentic for her tastes. The whole time the gun was on the table, which was only about a minute, she never took her eyes off it and never altered her cringing posture. Phil noticed this. After we had paid and we were out in the parking lot, Phil pulled out the gun and began jokingly threatening Faith with it, screaming "I want you, Faith!" and chasing her around the parking lot with the gun drawn as she squealed and ran away. The rest of us laughed, or pretended to. Phil stopped chasing Faith and the group reassembled for good-byes, as Christine's mom would soon be arriving to drive the girls back to their neighborhood. Much to Phil's and Adriana's chagrin, Christine's mom arrived early and there was no time for any good-night making out. Much to the rest of our delight, there was no need for an awkward good-bye.

Phil, Vic, and I began walking home along Water Street, next to the I-95 underpass, which we referred to as "under the bridge." This stretch was sketchy; many of the older kids hung out under the bridge to drink and do drugs and hook up, as we would in a few years. A lot of homeless people and a number of unsavory characters hung around there as well. But we stuck to the Water Street side, which was lined with abandoned factories, giant castles of concrete now boarded up, standing five or six stories high, eyesores that were once responsible for jobs for our grandparents' generation but now housed nothing but ghosts and dust. The black waters of the Delaware River trudged quietly along less than an eighth of a mile to our east; our homes and families were less than a quarter mile to our west.

We were not afraid, since this was a walk we each had done, later at night and without the benefit of friends, hundreds of times before. Besides, it was the quickest way to get home. We talked as we walked, an occasional car passing us, Phil swearing up and down that he had, in fact, had his hands up Adriana's shirt as they made out. While both Vic and I doubted this claim and said as much, I was too embarrassed to offer that I knew for certain that this was not true, because I watched Phil and Adriana make out for most of the night, hoping to collect any visuals that might possibly be useful for a masturbatory session later. A few blocks ahead of us, we saw a police paddy wagon turn onto Water Street, speeding along with its lights off, heading in our direction down the one-way street. "They were perfect," Phil said, "like this much," opening his hand wide to show the size of Adriana's boobs. The paddy wagon continued racing down the street, coming closer to us. "Swear to God—I swear on my mother. Jay, Vic, I swear on my mom I touched her tits." The paddy wagon was fifty feet away, and closing fast, speeding toward our direction.

Then the paddy wagon screeched to a halt just behind us. We turned to see that a cop had jumped out of the passenger door and drawn down on us, his pistol aimed squarely in our direction. His partner had run around from the driver's side and positioned himself through the open passenger window, standing behind the door and using it as a shield, gun also drawn and pointed at us. Two white guys, both in their mid-twenties, they were screaming, "Up against the fucking wall! Up against the fucking wall right now!" Before I knew what I was doing, I found myself voluntarily up against the fucking wall, standing against one of the abandoned factories, eyes closed, legs spread, arms planted firmly on the wall, just like I had seen in the movies, saying rapid-fire Our Fathers. To my right was Vic, in a similar posture, though I thought I could hear Hail Marys coming from him. To our left was Phil, standing, not facing the building but rather the cops. And he was talking. I did not see him reach into the waistband to pull out his fake gun, I only saw it in his hand. The cops' commands had changed to "Put the fucking gun down! Put the fucking gun down! Put the fucking gun down!" as Phil stood there, the gun lamely in his right hand, shining in the streetlight, as he gesticulated and pleaded, "It's fake! It's fake!" The cops were unmoved and continued to yell at it him to put the fucking gun down, to slowly put it on the ground, to put it down and get up against the wall, to put it down now. Phil acquiesced, slowly bent at his knees, put his fake gun on the ground, and positioned himself on the wall next to me and Vic. The cops moved to the gun and split up: one came over to Phil and put one hand on the back of his neck and ordered his hands behind his back, while the other picked the gun off the ground.

The first words I recognized were "You motherfuckers," followed shortly by, "It's a fake. It's a fucking toy." The cop who was holding Phil's neck let go, told him not to move, and took the gun from the other officer. He recognized that it was, as Phil had said, fake.

"You motherfucking cocksucker—you're lucky I don't slap the shit out of you. Unreal. Unfuckingreal." I did not move. Neither did Vic or Phil.

"Now get the fuck out of here. Now. Stupid fucking kids. Unfuckingreal. Stupid fucking kids."

And, yeah, we were. Stupid fucking kids.

Chapter Eleven

"Did I Ever Tell You About the Time I Got Arrested for Attempted Murder?"

For months, I grilled my parents while preparing for and writing this book. I sat down with each of them, together and separately, to mine their memories of any stories that I could use. I already knew of the big ones, the ones that I had heard over and over again while growing up and the ones that I lived through, but some were new to me. If there was anything that was funny, strange, or exciting that happened when I was a kid and I didn't know about it, I needed to know—*now*. I also interviewed them to fill in the details that I couldn't remember, either because I was too young to do so or because

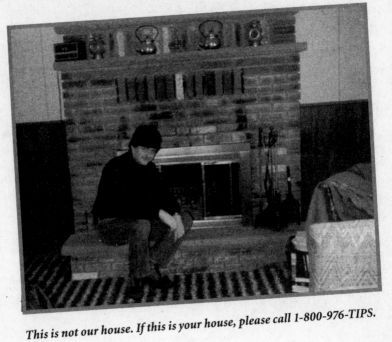

This is not our house. If this is your house, please call 1-800-976-TIPS.

I didn't realize what was really going on (as opposed to what I *thought* was going on). I was continually surprised during this part of process. Some of the things that I swore happened never actually did, or at least they did not in the way that I remembered them. It's amazing what the subconscious can suppress or alter when it really wants to.

I have no training in journalism (I have no training in anything, really, aside from maybe getting drunk and yelling at parked cars), but I worked very hard at getting these stories down. Okay, maybe not *very* hard, but certainly *reasonably* hard. After signing the book contract, I immediately went to Radio Shack and spent two hundred dollars on one of those little digital recorders. I figured I'd use it for interviews, which I would then download onto my laptop and use as my "primary source materials" as I hammered away on the book. This worked—for a little while, at least. I did get one interview on the recorder— a story about how my dad stole a car at fifteen and smashed it up—but then the batteries died. I forgot about the recorder for a few weeks until I started using it again not as an interview accessory but rather a way to record original songs of mine, which I would then email to friends.* Then I lost a lot of money gambling and so stopped writing songs, my inspiration having been sapped by the depression that comes with losing lots and lots of money. I'm not sure what happened to the recorder after that, but I think I lost it in a bar or something. Whatever.

The point is that what I lacked in training or technical know-how I made up for in tenacity. While preparing the book, I would call my family quite often, mostly out of the blue, to ask questions. They, particularly my mom and dad, were very patient with me, answering all my questions and queries, sometimes the same ones I had asked several times before while intoxicated or under the influence of marijuana. I ran up large phone bills spending hours over the weeks that I was working on this book talking to my family to get every last detail in, so that when I started writing these stories, they would come to me as naturally as though they had happened just yesterday.

One of my last steps in my research process was to write up a book outline, listing each chapter and providing a short synopsis of that chapter. I went over this with my parents, taking

---

* In addition to being a horrible writer, I'm also a really bad musician.

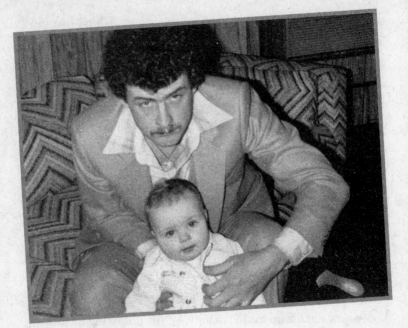

Getting ready to hit the town.

extra care to focus on the time frame when I was either not yet born or too young to remember, to ensure at any and all costs that I had *everything*. You only get to write a memoir once, I told them, and I wanted to make sure this was the definitive version.* After getting assurances from both my mother and my father that I did indeed have everything, I went full-steam ahead with the book. I would contact my parents with a question here and there, but I felt like I had control of the whole process. I even handed in the manuscript a full two weeks early, which

---

* I don't really believe this is true. I hope to milk my childhood for at least two, possibly three or four more books.

is unprecedented in the publishing industry.* When I did, I felt like a tremendous weight had been lifted off my shoulders. And it was time to party.

I left my home in New York to return to Philly for a few days of hanging out, binge drinking, and overeating. I had a great time, too, finally free from the book and another step closer to being a real writer. Joy. But after a few days, I had to return to New York. Whenever I'm in Philly, my dad always drives me to Thirtieth Street station, the main train station in Philadelphia, from where I take a train back up to NYC. Over the years this has developed into sort of a tradition. There are no great good-byes or pearls of wisdom or anything like that, just two guys driving in a truck, having a normal conversation. This most recent trip was no exception.

"So, done with the book, huh?" my dad asked.

"Yeah, all done. Thank God."

"That must feel good, to be done with all that work."

"Tell me about it."

About six full seconds of silence passed before my dad spoke again, saying offhandedly, "Oh—did I ever tell you about the time I got arrested for attempted murder?"

Um, what?

"Um, what?"

"Did I ever tell you about the time I got arrested for attempted murder?"

Hours of interviews, hundreds of questions, weeks and

---

* I have no idea whether this is true and it was early only in terms of my "final" deadline, after I missed my previous two deadlines. Whoops.

months of preparing and writing the book . . . no, I don't think he told me that he was arrested for attempted murder. "No, I think I would have remembered that."

"Oh, Jas," he chuckled, "that's a good one."

On the car ride to the train station, two weeks before my manuscript was due, *after* I had already handed it in, my dad told me about the time he was arrested for attempted murder.

So much for my investigative journalism.

Just before midnight on December 23, 1979, my dad left for work. He was working the midnight-to-eight shift that night on Pier 80, a large port on the Delaware River. While it was not an ideal shift for a new dad whose wife and young son were home alone so close to Christmas, a container ship had come in and needed to be unloaded. He got a call from the boss of his "gang," the term used to describe groups of longshoremen who worked together, and was asked to come in. So he didn't have much of a choice. Besides, union rules stipulated that December 24 was a holiday, which meant time-and-a-half pay. This overtime was much needed to offset some of the costs of raising a newborn, as well as the cost of the additional alcohol consumption that came with raising a newborn.[*]

Ships come from all over the world to the port of the Delaware River, which divides Pennsylvania and New Jersey. As a child, I'd be thrilled whenever my dad came home with coins from Europe, South America, even Africa that he had gotten

---

[*] I wasn't a crier, but more of a shrieker.

from visiting ships. This Christmas Eve ship came from China, and its cargo was giant containers filled with miscellaneous electronic devices: transistor radios, televisions, and the like. My dad's job was to roam the deck of the ship unlatching these containers, which had been tied down during transport so that they wouldn't shift as the ship traveled. Once they were un-latched, a giant crane would come down and lift the containers from the ship, placing them on the pier. They would be moved via forklift into storage and eventually be transported across the country.

My dad was working that night with a guy from the neigh-borhood, Billy Reynolds. Billy was a good guy, but a lunatic, always fighting, drinking, and getting into trouble. But of the three, fighting was his favorite, even though he was only five feet seven and about 160 pounds with a ten-pound sack in his hand.* But Billy, despite his reputation, was a good worker. Crazy guys are fun to be around—you never know when you're going to turn around to see them hanging off the side of a ship or taking a shit in the middle of the deck. The work can be boring, so a guy like Billy would spice it up by occasionally doing something stupid. And tough guys were ideal to work with. It's cold on the ship and the work is physical. The last thing you want is some-one up there with you complaining and lagging behind. After

---

* When Billy and his first wife divorced, she married a man from around the corner, a real bruiser named Joey Gilpatrick. She justified her choice of new husband by saying, "Well, Joey's the only guy around who can beat up Billy, so I really didn't have many options." This line has been repeated thousands of times and has become part of neighborhood lore. On a personal note, I can only hope that my wife chooses to marry me based on my ability to beat up her ex (or exes). I can't think of a better compliment.

all, once the cargo was properly unlatched, you could go home.

Or or or—if you finished early, you could hang around, still on the clock, soaking up that time-and-a-half pay (I mean, isn't this what being in a union is all about?), which is what my father and Billy decided to do on this night. They figured the job would take a full eight hours, so when they finished around 6:30 A.M., they decided to celebrate. And what better way to celebrate a job well done and Christmas Eve than with a drink?

Drinking on the job was not uncommon. You had your closet (or not-so-closet) alcoholics that would pack cases of beer in the trunks of their cars, retreating to the parking lot during downtime, of which there could be a lot. There was also a number of guys who would pack flasks and weren't afraid to bandy them about while working. As I said, "working longshore" is hard, unforgiving work. Sometimes one needed a pick-me-up. Sometimes one needed fifteen pick-me-ups. But now is not the time for judging.

My dad's and Billy's cocktail of choice on that Christmas Eve morning was something called a "shake-up," the main ingredient of which was grain alcohol. Though grain alcohol, which is 95 percent pure alcohol or 190 proof, was technically illegal, it was available.* More important, it was very, very efficient. A few sips of it and you didn't think about that cold December wind at

---

* This is another story in itself, since the grain alcohol was routinely stolen from a nearby liquor distillery plant. As it was told to me, all one had to do was walk into the compound, go to up a spigot, and pour the alcohol into an empty soda bottle. Though I have heard this from several people, I have no idea how this was possible. I can only assume that in the late '70s "security" hadn't really caught on yet.

all. The problem was that you didn't think about moving out of the way of the thousand-pound crane hook descending on you, either. The grain alcohol was too potent to be drunk straight, so it was often mixed with anything available to cut it—water, juice, soda—and shaken up, hence the "shake-up." This morning, orange juice was the mixer.

Whether my dad's original intention was only to have a few with Billy and then to head home at the end of the shift at eight is unknown. That's the beauty of alcohol, really, something that I have learned as well: each drink deepens the mystery and more dramatically alters the course of the day, the evening, or the night more than the previous one. In my mind I can see my dad and Billy, sitting in the small mechanics' shop, cluttered with tools and covered with grease, just off the pier on that morning, deciding to have one drink to help shake off the cold. A second would be poured because hey—it's Christmas Eve! A third because, well, why not? And a fourth would come just before clocking out, the proverbial "last one." But by that last one, my dad and Billy were feeling too good to end it there, so they left Pier 80 and drove into the neighborhood for a few more.

Billy's aunt and uncle owned a bar called Stevie & Karen's on the corner of Fourth and Moore streets. This was still technically in the neighborhood, but it was a bit on the outskirts, which means that the streets surrounding the bar were not the safest around. Because everything was so segregated—Irish here, Italians here, blacks here—when you stepped out of your element it was not unthinkable that you might run into some trouble. But this was of no concern to my dad and Billy on that Christmas Eve morning. When they arrived at the bar, hours before it was to open, they ascended the stairs on the side of the building leading to the apartment above where Billy's aunt and uncle lived. Billy turned on the charm and his uncle agreed to open the bar early so that he and my dad could have a few drinks and play some darts.

Meanwhile, back at home, my mother had no idea that my father was at a bar. It wasn't unusual for him to work late, so she wasn't bothered when he didn't get back after eight like he said he would. Besides, she was happy. Thrilled, even. She had her baby's first Christmas and had taken great pains to make it perfect. The gifts had all been wrapped, the Christmas tree decorated, and the stockings, which now read "Daddy" and "Mommy" instead of "Dennis" and "Kathy," along with a little one for "Jason," were hanging from the railing of the stairs. So even if Denny wanted to have a drink, let him have one. It *was* Christmas Eve and he *did* just work a bad shift, after all. It would take quite a lot to ruin this day for my mom.

Shortly after noon, the bar's regular opening time, business began to pick up. The regulars started filing in, a mix of retirees, loners, and alcoholics of all ages, as well as regulars guys looking to escape the holiday hubbub in their households. The mood, befitting the holiday spirit, was light and relaxed. While the world outside rushed to finish shopping or make preparations for a Christmas feast, time stood still inside the bar on Fourth and Moore.

It is my contention that in every drinking session, there are three critical points, three times during the session in which the drinker has a choice. If he chooses correctly, he will not tie on a load and instead will return home on his own volition safely and soberly. On the other hand, if he chooses incorrectly, he will probably have to be carried home by a bunch of guys he doesn't know who have most likely taken the liberty of relieving him of his wallet. In everyone's case, including my dad's on that Christmas Eve, the first critical point comes with the second drink. It's perfectly okay to have one drink, but when the second is offered and accepted, it begins a slippery slide toward a long night. Say no to that second drink and everyone walks away a winner. Say yes and your chance of doing something stupid or of something bad happening increases fivefold. When my dad agreed to have that second shake-up with Billy at work, Trouble wasn't exactly on his doorstep, but he was certainly up and awake and about to get in the shower.

The second critical point of my dad's day came when Billy suggested they go to his uncle's bar. Had he said no, my dad could have returned home with a nice buzz, but not too drunk to enjoy the rest of the day and spend it productively. Instead he accepted this invitation, and Trouble started the car and went out cruising. By the time of the third critical point of the drinking session they had already been in a bar for five hours. Billy suggested that instead of going out to grab lunch, they order in sandwiches. Welcome to Critical Point 3. To the casual drinker, Billy's offer might seem inconsequential. But to the experienced boozer like my father, this was key point in the day and the rest of the story. When Billy asked my father about having some sandwiches delivered, he more or less meant, "Look, you and I both know we're not leaving here anytime soon. Why don't we just have people bring us food so we can continue getting fucked up?" My father accepted. At that moment, Trouble saw Stevie & Karen's, thought it looked like a nice spot for a beer, and parked his car.

Cut to: At home, my mom was busy readying herself for Christmas Eve when the phone rang. It was my dad, asking if everything was all right, telling her that he was out but would be home soon. Annoyed but allayed, she carried on with her preparations. Trouble ordered a Bud, please.

Throughout the course of the day, my dad and Billy had made friends with many of the guys at the bar, and the whole afternoon turned into a chimerical montage of drinking, playing pool, laughing, drinking, playing darts, doing shots, and laughing. Neither Billy nor my dad had any concept of time until the six o'clock news came on, which meant dinnertime. With their heads swimming in booze, Billy and my dad got their things together to leave. They wore heavy clothes to work in order to brave the cold temperatures, thick Carhartt coveralls on top of their regular work clothes, which were layered upon long johns. They slowly, unsteadily climbed back into the heavy coveralls, which they had taken off when they first came into the bar. Finally suited up, they said their good-byes and headed outside.

It was now dark out. Snow covered the ground from a small storm just a day or two before. At the door of the bar, my dad and Billy shook hands and wished each other a Merry Christmas; it was the end of a hard shift and a fine day of drinking, and now it was time to return to family. Work, drink, family:

the holy trinity of the Irish Catholic, on the eve of the birth of Jesus Christ, no less.

As Billy turned away from my dad to head toward his car, he was blindsided—smacked in the face with a snowball, a direct hit. Hearing the thud of the snowball against Billy's head, my dad turned to see Billy stutter-step, gain his composure, and wipe the snow from his face, and take off running in the direction from which it came.

Second Street and the neighborhoods around it are very territorial. If you're white, you're not welcomed in the black neighborhood, and vice versa. This is not strictly a black-white issue and extends across all races and ethnicities—it would not be wise for an Irish kid to go walking around in the Italian neighborhood at night. This snowball was a "fuck you" to the white guys in the predominantly black neighborhood. Billy Reynolds, however, was not the guy to say "fuck you" to.

Billy and my dad gave chase. There ran after three guys, black kids maybe nineteen or twenty, just a few years younger than themselves. They followed them up Moore Street, heading toward Fifth Street. The kids made a right onto Fifth, and when my dad and Billy did the same, they saw that they were in for some trouble. A dozen black kids were standing on a stoop about halfway down the block.

Billy was a blowhard and never one to back down from a fight. But he had enough of a head on his shoulders to realize that things would not end well if too much aggression was used. As the dozen or so black kids approached my dad and Billy, there was only one viable thing to do to avoid getting jumped by all of them, which was to call out the guy who threw the snowball and ask for a one-on-one fight. "I got no problems," he said, "wit' none of you. I just want the guy who hit me in the face. I want him to be a man and own up."

Remarkably, this nearly always works. What Billy said follows a careful formula that has been crafted through generations of fighters when something is about to go down. "I got no problems wit' none of you" can roughly be translated to, "Let's think about this for second, because you know that I didn't do anything wrong here." It's about perspective: even though you or yours harmed me, I don't harbor any ill will toward your group. But by changing the dynamic to *I-You* (that is, I have no beef with you) versus *You-Me* (that is, you wronged me), it's much less accusatory and more conciliatory. I'm trying to be reasonable, and you should, too. Next is the call-out: I want only the guy who harmed me. This is another statement that is meant to show the use of reason and fairness, but it is slightly more aggressive because it places the ball squarely in the court of the person who committed the offense. He's now said, "I don't hate you guys, and I'm trying to be fair, so all I want is the guy who harmed me," a statement which by its very nature requires a response, one that will result in fight or flight. Finally, "I want him to be a man and own up" is the most aggressive of all, a direct challenge to the perpetrator's manhood. With this line, the result is almost guaranteed to be a fight, since if the offender refuses to "man up" to a challenge, especially in front of such a large contingent of his friends, which so outnumber the friends (in this case, friend) of his potential opponent, he will suffer a severe loss of respect, a commodity more valuable than anything else in the neighborhood.

I'd seen scenarios similar to this many times growing up, and the result was almost always the same: a situation that could have evolved into a brawl is averted and a fair fight between two guys, one the slighted, one the slighter, commences. This was no different, and the kid who hit Billy with the snowball stepped forward, a small kid, built remarkably like Billy. A circle tightened around the two of them—my father, rangy white guy, watching his friend Billy, rangy white guy, standing around with ten black guys who were not very happy to be with them.

More than half of street fights, probably even closer to two-thirds of them, don't have a clear winner. They usually follow a similar pattern. The fighters will square up, like boxers coming from their respective corners, and do some dancing in and out and throwing some feel-each-other-out punches. This is more show than anything, as one guy tries to out-intimidate the other with his aggressiveness and speed, and will last only a short while before the two guys grip each other up. If the two fighters fall to the ground, the fight will more than likely end with a winner, as one guy will get the advantage on top of the other guy and pummel him until he's pulled off. But if they stay standing up, they'll typically stay locked up and holding each other, throwing quick sneak punches, possibly head-butting, breaking off, and repeating the dancing and the gripping until it's broken up.

This particular fight was a strange sight. Whenever you're in a fight, real brawlers know that it's best to take off your shirt. If keep your shirt on and your opponent is able to get your shirt over your head, you're in some serious trouble. Not only will this cut off your vision, but it will incapacitate your arms by trapping them in the shirtsleeves above your head. So the other guy can basically tee off on you, his one hand holding the shirt over your head and his other blasting away, and if you're not dropped in three or four punches, you must have a metal plate in your head. Billy was a real brawler for sure and would have known this, being a veteran of dozens of fights. But he had his heavy longshoreman's gear on, which he could not step out of. These were both a blessing and a curse. While his coveralls lessened the impact of any punches thrown at his body, it limited his mobility and speed, causing him to move with the grace of the Stay Puft Marshmallow Man. Billy was a little guy whose toughness was based on his speed. Inhibited by the coveralls, he couldn't move like he needed to. While the full-body, inch-thick coveralls would have been great for a big guy whose MO was to grab and crush his opponent, it hampered Billy.

After a while of these two smaller guys locking up and throwing ineffective punches, it was apparent that this fight wasn't going anywhere. "All right, all right," called one of the black kids, who broke into the circle with a friend to separate his boy and Billy, and my dad followed them in.

"Fuckin' coveralls," Billy seethed when they were away from the group. "I'da killed that motherfucker if I didn't have these on."

"I know, I know," my dad offered, "but let's get the fuck out of here."

As they turned to walk away, Billy mumbling about how he could've killed the guy, he really could have, someone shouted "Hey!" from behind them. They turned to see one of the black kids approaching them.

"Yo, did you go to Southern?" he asked, looking at Billy, walking toward them. Southern was one of the local public high schools in South Philly and Billy had in fact gone there a few years before, but he had gotten thrown out and had not graduated. When he responded that yeah, he did go to Southern, the black kid said, "My man!" and extended his right hand for a handshake.

As he walked to Billy with his hand out for a shake, the kid raised his left hand, exposing the knife he was holding, and brought it quickly across Billy's right shoulder and chest. The knife ripped into Billy's coveralls, striking him in the upper chest. It continued along Billy's body, the blade making a quick ripping sound as it careened across his torso, tearing his clothes. The knife got caught up in the coveralls, dropped from the assailant's hand, and clanged down to the frozen, snow-dusted ground. Both Billy and my dad took off, racing back to the bar. The attacker and his gang fled in the opposite direction, taking cover in the side streets and the darkness.

It was on the sprint back to the bar that my dad heard the sound. It started softly at first, a muted hush, but then got louder, turning into hearty roar. Billy was laughing. He was, for certain now, a true lunatic.

And he continued laughing at the bar. The momentum of Billy's body falling backward and the thickness of the coveralls prevented the blade from going too deep, so the wound wasn't much—a simple cut on the upper part of his chest. While it might be a stretch to say that the thick longshoreman coveralls saved his life, it certainly saved him from a trip to the hospital and some stitches. The way that he carried on at the bar, you'd think that Billy had just hit the game-winning home run in a bar league softball game. Billy regaled the patrons with the story over another drink, contending over and over again, "No way he stabbed anybody before. That was his first time. He ain't never stabbed nobody before, because he doesn't know how to do it." This was way more excitement that my dad had signed on for when he agreed to do out for a drunk with Billy, and it was about time to call it an evening. As soon as he finished his beer.

Before he could finish that last beer, the thick wooden door of the bar swung wildly open and two police officers stormed in, guns drawn. "Nobody move! Hands in the air!" were their orders. They raced down the bar, checking the few patrons' faces. They stopped at my dad and Billy.

"This is them," one of the cops said, and placed them in handcuffs. My dad didn't speak, but Billy was irate. "What are you arresting me for! I was the one who was stabbed! What the fuck is your problem! *I* got stabbed!" He started stomping his feet like a child, repeating "*I* got stabbed!" and both he and my dad were put in a patrol car.

In the car, the cops were not very forthcoming to Billy's repeated pleas for an answer. Billy and my dad were working on a good cop–bad cop routine of their own, with Billy playing the role of screamer and my dad asking calmly what the problem was, why they were being held. Finally, one of the cops responded: "You're wanted for questioning about an attempted murder."

When a police officer drops the words *you, wanted,* and *attempted murder* in the same sentence, it's really time for some serious self-evaluation. That would have to be put on hold for a moment, because the patrol car pulled into the parking lot of Hahnemann Hospital, the same place my dad had gone years before when he broke his neck, and Billy and my dad were taken out of the car. They were led through the bowels of the hospital, still in cuffs, and up to the fourth floor, the Intensive Care Unit. They stopped at room 418 and were brought inside.

Sitting on the bed was a man of indeterminate age. He was conscious, but though the television was on he wasn't watching it. His face was the color of eggplant and swollen over. He had stitches on both of his eyelids and around his eyebrows; dried blood caked his mouth and forehead, and a large line of more stitches extended from just in front of his left ear down his check, ending at his jawline. His hands were swollen, and his arms were bruised and connected to an IV and other tubes. He looked blankly at the two cops and two prisoners standing before him.

The taller cop stepped forward, grabbed Billy's arm, and asked, "Is this him?"

The guy in the hospital bed looked at Billy, and then at my father, and then back at Billy.

"Nah, it ain't him. It's his brother."

Billy had two brothers; he was in the middle. His younger brother, Tommy, was the near complete opposite of Billy. Physically, he was a giant of a man, standing well over six feet two and 250 pounds. But he was also unlike Billy in disposition. Billy was a brawler, a lunatic; Tommy was a quiet, nice, churchgoing guy who kept to himself. If Billy's younger brother, Tommy, was the opposite of him, Billy's older brother, Pat, was a more amped-up version of Billy. Pat had the same small build as Billy, but everything else was turned up. Later, my dad explained it to me in the most concise way: "Billy'd beat you up, but Pat . . . Pat'd fuckin' kill you." And apparently, according to the beat-up man in the hospital bed, the authorities, and later a jury of his peers, that's what Billy's brother Pat had tried to do just a few hours before.

Pat was married to a woman named Linda. Linda got Pat a pretty crappy early Christmas present that year, when she told him on Christmas Eve, when his younger brother Billy and my dad were drinking at the bar, that she was having an affair. Pat had suspected as much, but that didn't lessen his anger any. He took a good shot at Linda, hitting her with a punch that sent her flying to the wall, and then grabbed his coat and headed out. Pat then paid a visit to the man who was making a cuckold of him, the same man who sat in the hospital bed before my dad and Billy. The cops were on the lookout for Pat when a tip came in that he was drinking at a bar at Fourth and Moore. Since Billy looked like Pat, Billy was picked up by the cops. My dad was picked up because he was with Billy. This where our case of mistaken identity comes from.

Both my dad and Billy were then taken to the precinct for questioning but later released, having no knowledge of what Pat did that day. My dad, now sober at this point, got a cab back to the bar, where his car was parked. He got home just before ten to find his wife, his parents, and her parents sitting around talking about the baby, who had just been put to bed. The room stood still and went silent when my dad walked through the entryway into the house. He sat down in his chair, took off his boots, let out a sigh, and said, "You wouldn't believe what happened to me today."

That was my first Christmas. A good one, I think.

Epilogue

Hooker Hunting

Whenever I go back home to Philly, I go hooker hunting.

Now I don't actually "hunt" the hookers, per se. I realize and appreciate the fact that hookers are women—wonderful, complex, yet misunderstood women—not game on some wildlife reserve. I'll be the first to concede that hooker hunting is not like hunting at all, really. I think I only call it "hooker hunting" because I like the alliteration.* Although it *is* kinda like a safari in that it is done at night and in a truck, but that's about where the similarities between the two end. Well, also, sometimes when push comes to shove, you have to shit in a bush. But we're getting off track here . . .

---

* Also, a group of my friends have taken to calling me "HH" ("Hooker Hunter"), which is imminently cooler than "HW" ("Hooker Watcher"). So *hooker hunting* it is.

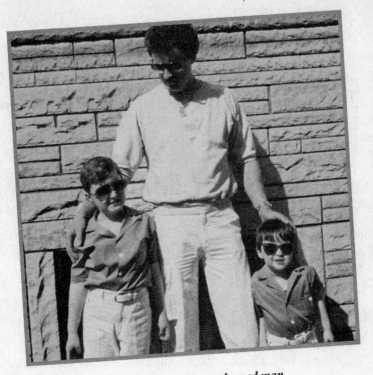

'Cause every girl's crazy 'bout a sharp-dressed man.

Instead, hooker hunting is more like *watching* than *hunting*. It's about observing; studying the hooker in her natural habitat. As an ornithologist might watch a rare robin or finch, so do I study the hookers of Philadelphia. I track movements, mannerisms, and social interaction. It is in this way that I have much in common with the scientists you see on the Discovery Channel, although I'm not sure if the scientists on the Discovery Channel secretly rub their private areas while watching their subjects. I don't watch much of the Discovery Channel, so I can't say for certain.

I'm not sure how I came up with the idea of hooker hunting, but like all of my best ideas, I'm guessing it was born from drunkenness and lust. I always find that whenever I'm visiting home in Philadelphia, I get very, very drunk. Don't get me wrong—I get very drunk in New York City, Boston, Los Angeles, and in pretty much every other city, town, or boat in America—but something about being in Philly and drinking with old friends puts me over the edge. And I'm not an economist, but I think this is also because in Philly I can plop down thirty dollars at a local watering hole and drink until I fall off the bar stool. Whereas in New York City, thirty dollars will get you a martini, but you probably won't have enough left over to tip the bathroom attendant.

Nor do I remember my first night hooker hunting. I can only assume it followed the pattern of later nights on the hunt—I get very drunk at a bar, spend all night unsuccessfully hitting on a woman, go to the local twenty-four-hour diner for some grub, then decide to go for a drive. And the hunt begins.

My vehicle of choice for the hunt is my dad's truck. No one drives in New York City, so I don't have a car (and there's the whole matter of how I'm broke). And I don't have a car waiting for me in Philly, so I have to use my dad's truck to get around. My dad got this truck a few years back and neither I nor my brother nor my sister have any doubt that he loves this truck more than any of us. If I had to come up with a list of the top five things my dad loves most, it'd go:

1. Marlboro Reds
2. The truck

3. Watching shows about serial killers

4. Coffee

5. Watching shows about nature

I can only hope that Dennis, Megan, and I make the top ten. But he really loves cereal, going to the bathroom, pizza, Marlboro Reds (again, just for the hell of it), and having a mustache, so I'm keeping my optimism within reason.

My dad has a gene that he did not pass on to either myself or my brother, the gene that is the basis for the complicated love between a man and his truck. When I look at my dad's truck, I see a mode of transportation that I can put a couch or a bookshelf in the back of. When my father looks at his truck, he sees everything that is right and good with being a man, the end result of hundreds of thousands of years of human evolution and mechanical development, the ultimate representation of the symbiotic relationship between man and machine. And he is happy.

He doesn't talk about the truck in affectionate terms. The truck does not have a name. It's not like he's out there washing and polishing it every Saturday afternoon. There's no cooing, there's no petting, tapping, patting, or any other silliness. Because that would be gay. And the truck itself is nothing special. It's not even really a truck, but rather one of those half-truck, half-SUVs that my dad decried as "stupid" for years before eventually buying one.* But the point I'm trying to get across

---

* I don't know why he did this; one thing my dad and I do not talk about is cars, since he spent his whole life working on them and I still sometimes get the gas and brake pedals confused. So we usually leave that topic alone.

is that though he loves it, it's not like it's a BMW or a Lexus or anything; it's just one of those average trucks. Not a piece of shit, but a plain, black, standard truck. And there's no physical manifestation for his love of this truck. If pressed about his feelings for his truck, he'd probably give a funny look and shrug it off. Love a truck? That's just stupid. Stupid.

And these are precisely the justifications I use when it's 4 A.M. and I'm drunk and I decide to drive his truck to look at hookers.

[Before I go any further, kids, please do not try this at home. Drunk driving is no laughing matter and I in no way support it. Unless you really don't have another option. Or you're not that drunk. Or you're doing it to impress a woman. But under any other circumstances than these, please don't drink and drive.]

It was a Saturday in December, a few weeks before Christmas. I was in Philly because I was doing "research" for this book, which, as mentioned, basically entailed asking awesome questions of my parents, like "So Mom, did you ever consider abandoning us, or perhaps abortion?" and "Dad, I'm going to say a word and I want you to say the first thing that comes to your mind: *methadone*. Thoughts?" After an exhausting day of work on the book (read: napping), I decided to meet some friends at our local bar, Mick-Daniel's. To say that Mick-Daniel's was my home away from home growing up would be a stretch, but I'm both lazy and not a good writer, so we'll have to stick with that.

I started working at the bar when I was about thirteen, washing dishes during the Friday and Saturday evening dinner hours. The money wasn't great but it was enough to get me by. But more important, the job was my first real experience with bar culture. And it was damn near love at first sight. I know this has something to do with how young I was at the time and how cool it was to tell my friends that I worked at a bar, even if I did only scrub grime off pots and pans. But there was something else. It was the excitement of the whole thing. It was watching how the bar transformed from 5 P.M., the start of my shift, to 10 P.M., the end of my shift. I'd watch the place slowly fill up with people, the lights getting dimmer and the music getting louder as the time passed; I'd see the smiles on the patrons' faces as friends showed up, watch them greet each other with handshakes, hugs, and pats on the back; I'd hear their bottles clink together in toasts, a sound drowned out by loud stories and laughter. In short, I was enthralled.

So it's no wonder that I return to Mick-Daniel's so often when I go home. I met my buddies Jimmy the Muppet and David there on this wintry night. Our intention was to take it easy—both Jimmy and David were hungover from the night before—but that plan went out the window around beer number 3. Then came beer number 4. Then beer number 6. Then beer number, um, 9? Then . . . sooner than we expected, the lights of the bar abruptly came on, signifying the end of the night. With many of the other patrons, we filed out of the bar on our way to the Oregon Diner, a twenty-four-hour place a few blocks away. It's not an unfamiliar scene to see groups of young people pouring out of the local bars at closing time, walking in formation to the diner, looking for a nightcap in the form of an open-face turkey sandwich or giant piece of apple pie.

I don't recall what food I went with that night. I usually start my postdrinking sober-up meal with French onion soup, then it's on to any combination of chicken fingers, broccoli bites, nachos, corn dogs, and pretty much any other food that will weaken my heart and/or colon. Whatever it was, the meal was quickly devoured as the three of us gulped it down like we were refugees. Soon we were tumbling back through the neighborhood to our homes, this time much more quietly, our drunken exuberance quelled by cheese, starch, and grease. Jimmy and David said good-bye and left me at the corner of my dad's street. I let myself in his house, grabbed his truck keys, and headed back out. It was time to go hunting.

[It's at this point that we must stop again to clear something up. Yes, I was drunk on this night. I would even say that yes, maybe I was even *very* drunk at certain points of the night. But I've found over the years that nothing sobers you up like a bowl of soup, a pound and a half of nachos, and four Sprites, so that by the time I started driving around, I was on the road to sobriety. Besides, what's the difference anyway? What are you—a fucking cop?]

Finding a parking spot is very difficult in my neighborhood, as it is in many cities. On the weekends, local public schools allow residents to park in their schoolyards to ease the burden of finding a spot. It was from one of these schoolyards that I took my dad's truck that night and started my drive.

The route was familiar to me by now, having been hooker hunting a dozen or so times before. Up Ritner to Broad, down Broad to Race, then making circles around the Center City area. One thing I picked up on these drives that I never before noticed about my hometown is how quickly and dramatically the streets of Philly can change. On one block, you'll find million-dollar town houses occupied by professionals, but three blocks north you'll drive by the same run-down houses that make nightly appearances on the news as crime scenes. I can offer no explanation for this, because, personally, if I'm dropping that much on a house, you'd better believe that the son of a bitch is going to have a pool and nary a crackhead within a twenty-mile radius. But this sudden and abrupt deterioration, I surmise, makes things easier for the working girls. You'll find them on the outskirts, or rather the *in*skirts, those blocks just within the nicer neighborhoods, hawking their wares. This is convenient. If they want, they can retreat into the sketchier parts of the neighborhood, but by stationing themselves on the nicer blocks their johns don't have to drive into the more dangerous areas.

What always surprises me is how normal the whole process appears. As I drove around and watched the girls casually stroll up to cars for a chat, I couldn't help but thinking, "Where are all the cops?" The girl will never get into the car right there, but instead instruct the driver to drive to a less crowded area and that's it. Simple, like two friends meeting up for a drive to the mall, not two strangers about to have sex for money.

I kept going in circles, checking out the scene, driving up, down, and around the streets of Center City Philadelphia. I'm not sure what compels me to do this. I have never been with a prostitute and am pretty sure I never will be. The combination of my Catholic guilt, my fear of disease, and probably most important, the potential embarrassment of getting caught will preclude me from such behavior for the rest of my life.* So it's not a sexual thing for me. It's more like the opposite of sexual, really; a morbid curiosity, a dark fascination. It's like watching a real live crime show on TV, but right before your eyes. I didn't stick around for too long—I usually don't—and after a few minutes and a couple of loops, I was on my way back home. The initial appeal wears off pretty quickly, especially since a friend had recently pointed out that police are supposed to patrol high-vice areas. Even though I'm usually sober by this point, or at least getting close to it, I think getting a DUI in an area known for prostitution might put my mother in a mental hospital. So I drove back home.

I took Broad Street south, making a left on Wolf Street. Driving down Wolf Street to Second Street, I'll come upon another night crawler, the junkie whore. You can catch them scurrying about the streets, an often terrifying spectacle, darting between parked cars and out into the street like stray cats. They are cracked-out women looking worse for the wear, ag-

---

* Unless I hit a major dry spell. But it's gotta be major—we're talking nothing for a solid two–three months. And not counting my bachelor party, of course, should I have one. I mean, duh.

ing a year for every month they use. Around the park between Sixth and Seventh streets, some of the junkies, when they see the truck coming down the street at 5 A.M., will come out of the darkness of the park or rush from their stoops onto the sidewalk and motion to the truck I'm driving, giving the universal mouth-hand sign for blow job, making clear in no uncertain terms that they're willing to offer sexual favors in exchange for cash or a fix. But I have neither, and consider myself just a spectator catching a half-drunk glimpse into the underside of urban nighttime. I was done for the night, tired, and I was going home. Also, getting a blow job from a junkie at 5 A.M. in your dad's truck, no matter how cool it may sound on paper, is just not a good idea. You know, so I've heard.

I started to grow precipitously tired on the drive home, but I was mere blocks away. As my eyelids grew heavier, I tightened my grip on the wheel and turned up the radio. Fortunately, the same spot I had vacated in the schoolyard a half hour before was open, so I pulled in. Had it been occupied, I could have parked somewhere else. I wasn't worried about my dad seeing that his truck had been moved. He's a late and heavy sleeper and I'm the opposite, so since I wake up before him I could always say that I took it in the morning out of the previous night's spot. Not a big deal.

I hastily pulled into the spot, shut the car off, and sat. I needed a minute before I went in. It was cold out, but the truck was nice and cozy. I just wanted one second to sit there and relax before I went in the house. So I sat back, took a deep breath, and closed my eyes.

* * *

When I woke up, at least an hour or two later, the sun was out. I was *freezing*. The windows had frosted over with my hot breath. I couldn't feel my nose, fingers, or toes. I could feel the cold deep, deep in my bones. As soon as I came to, my teeth started chattering uncontrollably. I didn't know what time it was. I knew only that it was really fucking cold and I really needed a bed. I left the truck, stumbled my way across the schoolyard, and made my way to my dad's house. The streets were still empty. After letting myself in, I stayed in the clothes I was wearing and bundled myself under the blankets and . . . *curtain*.

I awoke to a loud bang on the bedroom door. Not overly aggressive, but loud, assertive. It was my dad, calling my name and telling me to get up. I stretched and managed a meek "Hold on" as I kicked off my sneakers and took off my fleece to make it seem like I had a seminormal end to the night. When I opened the door, my dad had his back to me and was walking downstairs to the living room. I waited, curious, and then followed him as he reached the bottom of the stairs.

He sat down gingerly on his couch. In 2001, when he was forty-six, my dad got hurt at work. He now has four fused and six herniated vertebrae in his back and neck. Because of these injuries he's constantly in pain, but it's worse in the mornings. It takes him a good four hours, two pots of coffee, and his regimen of painkillers before he's able to leave the house to do anything productive.

"How was last night?" he asked me. His eyes were focused on the TV as he sipped his coffee.

"Good" was my reply. I knew he didn't want details and I didn't feel like going into them because I wanted to know what this wake-up call was all about. My mind was racing. Does he know that I took the truck? Did I hit something? Is it fucked up at all?

He leaned to one side in his chair and from his pocket pulled out the keys to his truck and threw them on the table between us.

Silence.

I waited, confused. He smoked.

He spoke, not turning from the television, "I went out to the truck this morning to get a pack of smokes and found these. In the ignition. With the lights on."

I froze.

He turned to look at me, finally, and through the cigarette smoke said, "Don't do that again."

At that moment, I gave up hooker hunting. I'd had a good run, but it was time.